(W)WILEY-BLACKWELL

This edition first published 2011. © 2011 by Blackwell Publishing Ltd

Blackwell Publishing was acquired by John Wiley & Sons in February 2007.
Blackwell's publishing program has been merged with Wiley's global Scientific,
Technical and Medical business to form Wiley-Blackwell.

Registered office: John Wiley & Sons Ltd, The Atrium, Southern Gate, Chichester,
West Sussex, PO19 8SQ, UK

Editorial offices: 9600 Garsington Road, Oxford, OX4 2DQ, UK
The Atrium, Southern Gate, Chichester, West Sussex,
PO19 8SQ, UK
2121 State Avenue, Ames, Iowa 50014-8300, USA

For details of our global editorial offices, for customer services and for
information about how to apply for permission to reuse the copyright material
in this book please see our website at www.wiley.com/wiley-blackwell.

Library of Congress Cataloging-in-Publication Data

Clinical diagnosis / edited by Phil Jevon.
    p. ; cm.
  Includes bibliographical references and index.
  ISBN 978-1-4443-3516-3 (pbk. : alk. paper)   1. Diagnosis, Differential.
2. Clinical medicine–Decision making.   3. Medical history taking.
I. Jevon, Philip.
  [DNLM: 1. Diagnostic Techniques and Procedures. WB 141]
  RC71.5C38 2010
  616.07'5–dc22

                                                        2010040964

A catalogue record for this book is available from the British Library.

This book is published in the following electronic formats: ePDF 9781444340037;
Wiley Online Library 9781444340051; ePub 9781444340044

Set in 9/11 pt Palatino by Aptara® Inc., New Delhi, India

Printed and bound in Malaysia by Vivar Printing Sdn Bhd

1   2011

Contents

Contributors List

Kathryn Blakey, MBBS nMRCGP
General Practice vocational training scheme
Birmingham
West Midlands

Yonas Mhando, MD
GPST Trainee, Northern Deanery;
Formerly Clinical Teaching Fellow & Honorary Clinical Lecturer University of Birmingham & Manor Hospital, Walsall, West Midlands

Dev Mohan Gulur, MBBS, MRCS
SpR in Urology, Mersey Rotation

Phil Jevon, RN, BSc (Hons), PGCE Resuscitation
Officer/Clinical Skills Lead
Manor Hospital, Walsall

Dev Mittapalli, MBBS, MRCS, PGCME
SpR in General Surgery, East of Scotland (Dundee) Surgical Rotation, and Honorary Clinical Lecturer at the University of Birmingham

Michael Parry, BSc (Hons), MBChB, MRCS
Specialist Registrar, Severn Deanery and Clinical Research Fellow, University of Bristol

Gareth Walters, BSc (Hons), MBChB MRCP (UK), MRCP (London), FHEA, MinstLM, LCGI
Specialist Registrar in Respiratory and General Medicine, West Midlands Rotation, and Honorary Clinical Lecturer, University of Birmingham

Yi-Yang Ng, MBChB, MRCS, AHEA, PGCME
GP Registrar, Dartford, Kent Sussex and Surrey Deanery previously Clinical Teaching Fellow, Manor Hospital Walsall, West Midlands and Honorary Clinical Lecturer University of Birmingham

Foreword

As nursing progresses in terms of skill set and competencies focusing on patient pathways, there is a requirement to support professionals with up to date and relevant tools to support them. Clinical diagnosis can be complex and we know that timely and effective clinical diagnosis delivers optimum outcomes for patients.

This book is designed as a practical guide to support nurses in their decision making. It is well written and has had relevant clinical experts contributing chapters. It is comprehensively written and follows a systems approach providing a logical structure.

The editor must be commended for his foresight in developing this book and I am confident that many nurses will use this excellent guide in supporting their decision making and improving outcomes for patients. I am delighted to recommend this book and wish that this had been available to me many years ago!

Sue Hartley
Director of Nursing and Governance
Walsall Hospitals NHS Trust

An Overview to Clinical Diagnosis

1

Phil Jevon

LEARNING OUTCOMES

At the end of this chapter, the reader will be able to:

❏ list the objectives of history taking,
❏ discuss establishing a rapport with the patient,
❏ describe the importance of effective listening skills,
❏ discuss the sequence of history taking,
❏ provide an overview to clinical examination,
❏ discuss the symptoms of disease and
❏ outline the role of tests and investigations.

INTRODUCTION

The term 'clinical' originates from the Greek word *klinike* meaning bedside (Soanes & Stevenson 2006). Diagnosis, which originates from the Greek word *diagignoskein* meaning distinguish or discern, can be defined as the identification of the nature of an illness or other problem by examination of the symptoms (Soanes & Stevenson 2006).

History taking (discussing the patients' complaints with them) and clinical examination, together with performing or ordering relevant investigations, are essential for clinical diagnosis (Cox & Roper 2006). Despite the advances in modern diagnostic tests, history taking and clinical examination remain

Clinical Diagnosis, 1st edition. Edited by Phil Jevon.
© 2011 Blackwell Publishing Ltd.

fundamental in determining the most appropriate treatment (if any) for the patient. History taking is considered one of the most important aspects of patient assessment and is being increasingly undertaken by nurses (Crumbie 2006).

History taking and clinical examination require a structured, logical approach to ensure that all the relevant information is obtained and that nothing important is overlooked. History taking and clinical examination skills are difficult to acquire and, above all, require practice (Gleadle 2004).

The aim of this chapter is to provide an overview to clinical diagnosis.

OBJECTIVES OF HISTORY TAKING

History taking is like being a detective: 'searching for clues, collecting information without bias, yet staying on track to solve the puzzle' (Clark 1999). It is important for making a provisional diagnosis; clinical examination and investigations can then help to confirm or refute it. The history will provide information about the illness as well as the disease; the illness is the subjective component and describes the patient's experience of the disease (Shah 2005a). A carefully taken medical history will provide the diagnosis or diagnostic possibilities in 78% of patients (Stride & Scally 2005).

The objectives of history taking are to

- establish a rapport with the patient,
- elicit the patient's presenting symptoms,
- identify signs of disease,
- make a diagnosis or differential diagnosis and
- place the diagnosis in the context of the patient's life.

ESTABLISHING A RAPPORT WITH THE PATIENT

Establishing a rapport with the patient is essential. Rapport can be defined as the ability to being on the same wavelength and to connect both mentally and emotionally with a person, thus promoting trust and mutual respect (Moulton 2007). If the patients believe that they are getting the nurse's full attention, they are more likely to try to accurately answer questions and recall past events.

To establish a rapport and to put the patient at ease, it will be helpful to start the examination/interview by considering such issues as the following:

- *Physical distance between the patient and the nurse.* This can have a direct impact on rapport (Kaufman 2008). It is important to get the balance right between not being too close to the patient, which could be interpreted as over-familiarity, and not being too far from the patient, for example behind a large desk.
- *Positive initial contact.* Shake the patient's hand while introducing yourself.
- *Privacy.* Reassure the patient that their privacy and dignity will be maintained.
- *Patient's name.* Establish how the patient would like to be addressed (forename or surname). It is particularly important to know the patient's name (Clark 1999).
- *Patient's physical comfort.* Ensure that the patient is in a comfortable position, and position yourself so that the patient is not sitting at an awkward angle.
- *Confidentiality.* Reassure the patient that all their information will be treated as confidential.
- *Posture.* Avoid standing up, towering over the patient; ideally, sit down at the same level as the patient (Figure 1.1).
- *Effective communication skills* (Box 1.1). In particular, allow time to listen to what the patient is saying and avoid appearing to be rushed.
- *Appropriate language.* Appropriate language and understanding are important aspects of history taking; as the patient may not understand a particular word or phrase, always have an alternative available, for example 'phlegm' in place of 'sputum'. Ensure that the patient understands the question or any information given to them (Shah 2005b). Also, if the patient does not understand English, communicate through an interpreter, if possible.

IMPORTANCE OF EFFECTIVE LISTENING SKILLS

As mentioned above, communication is an essential part of history taking. Active listening is particularly important (Kaufman

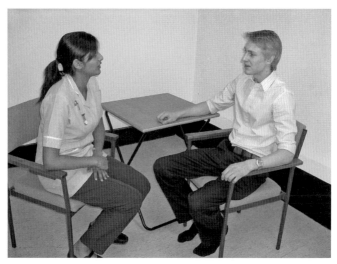

Figure 1.1   It is important to establish a rapport with the patient.

2008), especially when trying to establish a reliable and accurate clinical diagnosis. There is good evidence linking effective communication with improved patient outcomes (Gask & Usherwood 2002).

The SOLER framework has been suggested by Egan (2007) to reinforce the non-verbal elements of active listening (Box 1.2).

Box 1.1   Effective communication skills involved in history taking (Shah 2005a)

- Opening and closing a consultation
- Using open and closed questions
- Using non-verbal language
- Active listening
- Showing respect and courtesy
- Showing empathy
- Being culturally sensitive

Box 1.2   The SOLER framework for non-verbal components of active listening (Egan 2007)

Sit *S*quare onto the patient.
Adopt an *O*pen position.
*L*ean slightly forward.
Maintain *E*ye contact.
Adopt a *R*elaxed posture.

SEQUENCE OF HISTORY TAKING

The following sequence of history taking is recommended (Ford *et al.* 2005):

- introduction;
- presenting complaint and history of current illness;
- systemic enquiry;
- past medical history;
- drugs;
- allergies;
- family history;
- social and personal history;
- patient's ideas, concerns and expectations.

Introduction

It is important to introduce yourself to the patient, for example stating your name and position. Confirm the identity of the patient: ask their name and how they prefer to be addressed. Consent should then be sought for history taking and clinical examination.

Presenting complaint and history of current illness

By far the most important part of history taking and clinical examination is the history of the patient's presenting complaint and history of current illness; the information elicited usually helps to make a differential diagnosis and provides a vital insight into the features of the complaints that the patient is particularly concerned about (Gleadle 2004).

Therefore, a large part of history taking involves asking questions concerning the patient's presenting complaint(s) to establish the main symptom(s). The objective is to obtain a chronological account of the relevant events, including any interventions and outcomes, together with a detailed description of the patient's main symptoms (Ford *et al.* 2005).

Ask the patient to describe what has happened to bring them to the hospital or to make them seek medical help. Their narrative will provide important clues as to the diagnosis and their perspective of their illness. Do allow the patient ample time to do this; it is important not to interrupt. Clinicians often interrupt to enquire about the first issue raised by the patient (Kaufman 2008). However, the first issue may not actually be the main problem concerning the patient, and once the clinician has interrupted, the patient often does not introduce new issues (Gask & Usherwood 2002).

Short responses such as 'Please tell me more' and 'Go on' will encourage the patient to elaborate. Once the presenting complaint has been established, it must be carefully evaluated in detail (Shah 2005a):

- What was the start date/time?
- Who noticed the problem (patient, relative, caregiver, health care professional)?
- What initial action did the patient take (any self-treatment)? Did it help?
- When was medical help sought and why?
- What action was taken by the health care professional?
- What has happened since then?
- What investigations have been undertaken, and what are planned?
- What treatment has been given?
- What has the patient been told about their problem?

Systemic enquiry

Systemic enquiry is a series of questions related to the bodily systems which allows more information that can be linked to the presenting complaint to be obtained; considered a safety net,

Table 1.1 Units of alcohol in common drinks (Department of Heath 2008)

1 pint of ordinary strength beer = 2 units
1 pint of ordinary strength cider = 2 units
1 pub measure of spirit = 1 units
1 glass of wine = 2 units
1 alcopop = 1.5 units

it reduces the risk of missing an important symptom or disease (Shah 2005b).

However, systemic enquiry can cause confusion and misdirect the clinician if the patient has multiple symptoms or is garrulous. It should therefore be undertaken systematically and carefully: a suggested 'checklist approach' is detailed in Table 1.2.

It is standard practice to start with the most relevant system(s) to the presenting complaint; for example if the patient presents with chest pain, questions about the cardiovascular and respiratory systems should initially be asked (Shah 2005b). The depth of questioning will depend on personal experience, the individual patient, their presenting complaint, the situation and circumstances.

Past medical history
It is useful to establish the patient's past medical history because of the following:

- If they have a longstanding disease, there is a strong possibility that any new symptom could relate to it.
- It could help with making the correct diagnosis.
- It is helpful when establishing the most appropriate treatment for the patient.

Ask the patient if they have ever had any serious illness or been admitted to hospital previously or had surgery. It is a usual practice to record whether they have suffered from/suffer from any of the following illnesses (Gleadle 2004):

- jaundice,
- anaemia,

Table 1.2 Systemic enquiry

General
- Well/unwell
- Weight gain or loss
- Appetite good or poor
- Fevers
- Sweats
- Rigours

Cardiovascular
- Chest pain
- Breathlessness
- Orthopnoea
- Paroxysmal nocturnal dyspnoea
- Ankle swelling
- Palpitations
- Collapse
- Exercise tolerance
- Syncope

Respiratory
- Cough
- Shortness of breath
- Haemoptysis
- Sputum
- Wheeze
- Pleuritic pain

Nervous system
- Headaches
- Fits
- Blackouts
- Collapses
- Falls
- Weakness
- Unsteadiness
- Tremor
- Visual and sensory disorders
- Hearing disorder

Gastrointestinal
- Nausea
- Vomiting
- Diarrhoea
- Abdominal pain
- Mass
- Rectal bleeding
- Change in bowel habit
- Dysphagia
- Heartburn
- Jaundice
- Anorexia/weight loss

Musculoskeletal
- Weakness
- Joint stiffness
- Joint pain/swelling
- Hot/red joints
- Reduced mobility
- Loss of function

Genitourinary
- Dysuria/urgency
- Haematuria
- Frequency
- Nocturia
- Urinary incontinence
- Urethral/vaginal discharge
- Menstrual cycle
- Sexual function

Skin
- Rash
- Lumps
- Itch
- Bruising

- tuberculosis,
- rheumatic fever,
- diabetes,
- bronchitis,
- myocardial infarction/chest pain,

- stroke,
- epilepsy,
- asthma and
- problems with anaesthesia.

Drugs

Obtaining a drug history is helpful because of the following:

- Side effects of drug therapy could be the cause of the patient's presenting complaint.
- Before starting or adjusting drug treatment, it is important to be aware of what the patient is already taking; for example old drug therapy could be ineffective or may interact with new drug therapy.

Establish if the patient is taking any of the following (Shah 2005b):

- prescription drugs;
- over-the-counter drugs, that is, drugs bought without a prescription, for example aspirin;
- herbal or 'natural' treatments;
- illegal or recreational drugs.

If the patient is taking medications, establish the dose, route of administration, frequency and period of time they have been taking the medications. The possibility of non-compliance with prescription drugs should also be considered.

The patient may be unsure what drugs they are taking. Under these circumstances, it is worthwhile using the medical history and asking them if they are taking any treatment for each problem; for example 'Do you take anything for your arthritis?' (Shah 2005b).

In addition, if the patient knows what drugs they are taking, it can be helpful to ask them what they are taking the drugs for, because this may sometimes provide helpful additional information related to the patient's illnesses (Shah 2005b).

Allergies

An accurate and detailed description of any allergic responses the patient may have to drugs or other allergens should be recorded; in particular, the patient should be asked whether they are allergic to penicillin. If the patient has an allergy, try to determine what actually happened, in order to differentiate between an allergy and a side effect (Shah 2005b); 'side effect' refers to an effect of a drug which is not that which the doctor and the patient require, while 'allergy' is a term usually used to describe an adverse reaction by the body to a substance it has been exposed to (Marcovitch 2005). The wearing of a 'medic-alert' bracelet and the reason for doing so should be noted.

Family history

It is important to establish the diseases that have affected the patient's relatives because there is a strong genetic contribution to many diseases (Gleadle 2004).

Shah (2005b) recommends the following approach to taking a family history:

- Ascertain who has the problem: is it a first- or second-degree relative?
- Determine how many family members are affected by the problem.
- Clarify what exactly the problem is: for example 'a problem with the heart' could be several things – hypertension, ischaemia, valve problems and the like. Be exact as to the nature of the problem because several family members may have 'heart problems', but they may be completely different and, therefore, not relevant to the patient's particular problem.
- Determine at what age the relative developed the problem; obviously, early presentation is more likely to be important than one presenting later in life.
- Ascertain if the patient's parents are still alive and, if not, at what age they died and the cause of death.

Social and personal history

Social history
It is important to understand the patient's social history: their background, the effect of their illness on their life and on the lives of their family (Gleadle 2004).

- *Marital status and children*. Ask whether they are married/have a partner and whether they have children. This is particularly important if the patient is frail and elderly because it will help to ascertain whether the family will be able to look after them if required (Cox & Roper 2006).
- *Occupation*. Establish the patient's occupation (or previous occupation if they have retired). As certain occupations are at risk of particular illnesses, a full occupational history is paramount (Gleadle 2004); for example construction workers may suffer from asbestos-related diseases. Some occupations can be affected by certain diseases; for example a lorry driver diagnosed with epilepsy will need to give up his job (Cox & Roper 2005).
- *Living accommodation*. Ascertain where the patient lives and the type of accommodation they live in, for example a bungalow, a house with an upstairs bathroom or a block of flats, as this could be pertinent as both a contributing factor to their presenting complaint and a consideration when discharging the patient.
- *Travel history*. Nowadays, with illnesses such as SARS (severe acute respiratory syndrome) and avian flu, a travel history is essential (Shah 2005b), particularly if infection is suspected.
- *Patient's hobbies/interests*. Having a knowledge of these allows a clinician to understand the patient better and to determine what is important to them (Shah 2005b).

Smoking and alcohol
It is important to establish the patient's current and past smoking and alcohol history because both are implicated in many illnesses:

- *Smoking*. Ask the patient if they smoke; if they do, confirm details of what they smoke, that is, cigarettes, cigars or a pipe, including the quantity that they smoke and how long they have been a smoker; if the patient does not smoke but has smoked previously, again confirm the details of what they smoked, that is, cigarettes, cigars or a pipe, the quantity that they smoked, for how long they smoked and when they gave it up.

• *Alcohol.* Ask the patient if they drink alcohol; use the standard unit as a measure (Table 1.1). As there is a tendency to underestimate alcohol intake, separate weekday and weekend intake should be established, together with any history of binge drinking (do not forget to include wine taken with meals, as this is often forgotten; Shah 2005b). Adopt a non-judgemental approach, but get to the point, for example by asking, 'How much alcohol do you normally drink?' or, if there is no clear answer, 'How much did you drink in the last week/fortnight?' (Shah 2005b).

Patient's ideas, concerns and expectations

An appropriate and sound history-taking technique will help to identify the patient's ideas, concerns and expectations. Effective communication techniques (listed in Box 1.1) are paramount. The most common cause of patient dissatisfaction following a consultation is a failure in communication (Ford *et al.* 2005). To help to avoid this situation, it would be helpful to do the following:

• Thank the patient for their cooperation (Shah 2005b).
• Ask the patient if there is anything else they would like to say. This allows the patient a final opportunity to add any additional information (Lloyd & Craig 2007).
• Provide a short summary outlining the patient's problem or symptoms – this will help to confirm a mutual understanding, reducing the risks of a misunderstanding; it also allows the patient to clarify details and make any corrections if necessary (Moulton 2007).

AN OVERVIEW OF CLINICAL EXAMINATION

Having completed history taking, a differential diagnosis will be possible, which will help to direct the focus of clinical examination (Ford *et al.* 2005). A suggested approach to clinical examination will now be described.

Preparation

- Obtain the patient's consent (Nursing and Midwifery Council [NMC] 2004).
- Assemble any necessary equipment and aids required for the examination.
- Adhere to local infection control protocols as appropriate; for example wear appropriate clothing and wash and dry hands.
- Ensure privacy: screen the bed or the couch.
- Consider the need for a chaperone who should be of the same gender as the patient (Thomas & Monaghan 2007). The patient has a right to request a chaperone when undergoing any procedure or examination; where intimate procedures or examinations are required, the nurse should ensure that she is aware of any cultural or religious beliefs or restrictions the patient may have which prohibit this being done by a member of the opposite sex (NMC 2008).
- Clear the left side of the bed (the right side of the patient) – always perform the examination from the left side of the bed (Cox & Roper 2006), unless left-handed in which case approach from the right, as this will provide the nurse with a feeling of control over the situation (Thomas & Monaghan 2007).
- While exposing the area that needs to be examined, avoid embarrassing the patient; ensure that there are no draughts, and close any open windows if necessary. It is important that the patient does not get cold during the examination: shivering will cause muscle sounds which will interfere with auscultation (Ford *et al.* 2005).
- Position the patient appropriately on the couch/bed: initially, this will be sitting at an angle of 45° for the examination of the cardiovascular system. The position will usually be changed for other aspects of the examination; for example for the examination of the abdomen, the patient will need to be in a supine position. Sometimes the patient position will be determined by their condition; for example if they are very

breathless, they will probably need to sit at $90°$; if they are unconscious, they will be flat throughout the examination.

- Ensure that the hands are warm before examining the patient: palpating using cold hands can result in the contraction of abdominal muscles, impairing the examination (Ford *et al.* 2005).

Procedure for clinical examination

The procedure for clinical examination can be broken down into bodily systems. These bodily systems should be examined in turn:

- cardiovascular system;
- respiratory system;
- gastrointestinal system;
- genitourinary systems;
- neurological system;
- skeletal system;
- ear, nose and throat.

Examination of each system should encompass the following (Gleadle 2004):

- inspection (looking),
- palpation (feeling),
- percussion (tapping) and
- ausculation (listening).

Although described separately in different chapters, the examination routines for each system should not be considered as entirely separate entities: when examining several systems at once, a single fluid routine should be used throughout the clinical examination.

Following clinical examination

Following clinical examination, it is important to

- thank the patient for their help and co-operation;
- invite and answer any questions they may have;
- ensure that the examination routine is formally closed so that the patient knows that it has finished;
- leave the patient in a comfortable position and not exposed;
- ensure appropriate documentation (NMC 2004, Chapter 9).

SYMPTOMS OF DISEASE

A symptom can be defined as an indication of a disease or disorder noticed by the patient (a sign is an indication of a particular disease or disorder that is observed during clinical examination; McFerran & Martin 2003). A comprehensive and effective history-taking technique will help to elicit the patient's symptoms.

Each symptom must be methodically analysed. It is important to encourage the patient to describe their symptoms in an expansive manner (Kaurfman 2008). A number of frameworks have been developed to help this process.

Ford *et al.* (2005) suggest the TINA system approach:

- Timing – onset, duration, pattern and progression.
- Influences – precipitating, aggravating and relieving factors.
- Nature – character, site, severity, radiation and volume.
- Associations – any other associated signs and symptoms.

Perhaps a more helpful framework is the mnemonic PQRST suggested by Zator Estes (2002):

- Provocation and Palliation – what exacerbates and what relieves the symptom; this information in particular can provide important clues to assist in diagnostic decision-making (Kaufman 2008).
- Quality – how the symptom appears to the patient.
- Region and Radiation – ascertaining the region and radiation can again help with diagnosis.
- Severity – a scale of 0–10 is usually used to describe the severity of the pain or the symptom (Kaufman 2008).
- Timing – it is helpful to establish when the symptom started, its timing during the day, its pattern and consistency and whether it is continual or intermittent (Kaufman 2008).

TESTS AND INVESTIGATIONS

Try to follow the sequence of history taking, then clinical examination and then tests and investigations when seeing a patient; a common mistake is to rush into investigations before considering the history or clinical examination (Stride & Scally 2005).

When ordering tests and investigations, it is easy to mindlessly order a whole range of them. However, there are many problems with this approach (Stride & Scally 2005):

- Investigations cannot be used in isolation – is the X-ray finding or blood test result relevant or an incidental finding?
- Investigations can be inaccurate – there can be problems with the technique, reagents or interpretation of the findings.
- Investigations pose risks – radiation exposure, unnecessary further procedures and so on.
- Investigations can be costly, to the patient and to society.

Therefore, after history taking and clinical examination, order or perform tests and investigations relevant to the case (Beasley *et al.* 2005).

CONCLUSION

This chapter has provided an overview to clinical diagnosis. The objectives of history taking have been listed, and how to establish a rapport with the patient has been described. The sequence of history taking, together with symptoms of the disease, has been discussed. Furthermore, an overview to clinical examination has been provided.

REFERENCES

Beasley, R., Robinson, G. & Aldington S (2005) From medical student to junior doctor: the scripted guide to patient clerking. *Student BMJ* **13**, 397–440.

Clark, C. (1999) Taking a history. In: Walsh, M. (ed.) *Nurse Practitioners: Clinical Skills and Professional Issues.* Butterworth Heinemann, Oxford.

Cox, N. & Roper, T. (2005). *Clinical Skills: Oxford Core Text*. Oxford University Press, Oxford.

Crumbie, A. (2006) Taking a history. In: Walsh, M. (ed.) *Nurse Practitioners: Clinical and Professional Issues*, 2nd edn. Butterworth Heinemann, Edinburgh, UK, pp. 14–26.

Department of Health (2008) http://www.dh.gov.uk

Egan, G. (2007) *The Skilled Helper*. BrooksCole/Thomson Learning, Belmont, CA.

Ford, M., Hennessey, I. & Japp, A. (2005) *Introduction to Clinical Examination*. Elsevier, Oxford.

Gask, L. & Usherwood, T. (2002) ABC of psychological medicine. *British Medical Journal* **324** 1567–1569.

Gleadle, J. (2004) *History and Examination at a Glance*. Blackwell, Oxford.

Kaufman, G. (2008) Patient assessment: effective consultation and history taking. *Nursing Standard* **23** (4), 50–56.

Lloyd, C. & Craig, S. (2007) A guide to taking a patient's history. *Nursing Standard* **22** (13), 42–48.

Marcovitch, H. (2005) *Black's Medical Dictionary*, 41st edn. A & C Black, London.

McFerran, T. & Martin, E. (2003) *Mini-dictionary for Nurses*, 5th edn. Oxford University Press, Oxford.

Moulton, L. (2007) *The Naked Consultation: A Practical Guide to Primary Care Consultation Skills*. Radcliffe, Abingdon, UK.

Nursing and Midwifery Council (2004) *The NMC Code of Professional Conduct: Standards for Conduct, Performance and Ethics*. Nursing and Midwifery Council, London.

Nursing and Midwifery Council (2008) *Chaperoning*. http://www.nmc-uk.org (accessed 26 January 2008).

Shah, N. (2005a) Taking a history: introduction and the presenting complaint. *Student BMJ* **13**, 309–352.

Shah, N. (2005b) Taking a history: conclusion and closure. *Student BMJ* **13**, 353–396.

Soanes, C. & Stevenson, A. (2006) *Concise Oxford English Dictionary*, 11th edn. Oxford University Press, Oxford.

Stride, P. & Scally, P. (2005) Better ways of learning. *Student BMJ* **13**, 353–396.

Thomas, J. & Monaghan, T. (2007) *Oxford Handbook of Clinical Examination and Practical Skills*. Oxford University Press, Oxford.

Zator Estes, M. (2002) *Health Assessment and Physical Examination*, 2nd edn. Delmar Cengage Learning, New York.

2 | Clinical Diagnosis of Symptoms Associated with the Respiratory System

Gareth Walters

The aim of this chapter is to understand the clinical diagnosis of symptoms associated with the respiratory system.

LEARNING OUTCOMES
At the end of this chapter, the reader will be able to discuss the clinical diagnosis of the following symptoms associated with the respiratory system:

- ❑ acute breathlessness,
- ❑ cough,
- ❑ haemoptysis,
- ❑ digital clubbing and
- ❑ inspiratory stridor.

ACUTE BREATHLESSNESS
Breathlessness (or dyspnoea) is defined as difficulty in breathing (Marcovitch 2005) or the uncomfortable awareness of one's own breathing (Chapman *et al.* 2009). The word 'dyspnoea' derives from the literal Greek translation of *dys* meaning 'difficulty' and

Clinical Diagnosis, 1st edition. Edited by Phil Jevon.
© 2011 Blackwell Publishing Ltd.

pnoia meaning 'breathing'. Breathlessness can be a subjective sensation, that is, reported by the patient. For example, a patient might suggest that they feel 'short of puff' when they climb the stairs. However, breathlessness can also be objectively assessed by others. For example, a patient may be *seen to have* a high respiratory rate (>20 breaths/min) on walking to the bathroom.

It is important to note that a patient who *feels* breathless may not necessarily appear to *be* breathless on examination. Acute respiratory distress describes an extreme state, where poor oxygenation means that even a rapid breathing rate is insufficient to maintain adequate tissue oxygen levels (tissue hypoxia). The patient requires a rapid assessment to quickly identify the cause of acute breathlessness.

Acute breathlessness is one of the most common reasons for admission to hospital (Cox & Roper 2005) and can represent a broad variety of diseases. Patients will present to accident and emergency, or be admitted via emergency ambulance on a daily basis, with acute breathlessness and acute respiratory distress. Additionally, patients on the wards may become acutely breathless following deterioration in their condition or the sudden onset of a new pathology such as pulmonary embolism.

Causes

There is a broad spectrum of diseases that cause acute breathlessness, but a handful of very common causes. These are listed in Table 2.1. Most of the potentially serious and life-threatening cardiac and respiratory disorders present with acute breathlessness.

The underlying disease dictates the pathophysiology of abnormal breathing, but in most cases, the breathlessness is caused by the following:

- lack of oxygen reaching the capillaries in the lung (hypoxia) because of lung or pulmonary vascular disease;
- lack of oxygen reaching the tissues of end organs such as the heart muscle, kidneys or skeletal tissue (tissue hypoxia).

Table 2.1 Causes of acute breathlessness.

Respiratory causes	Common
	Acute pulmonary embolism
	Pneumothorax
	Pneumonia
	Exacerbation of COPD
	Acute severe asthma
	Massive pleural effusion
	Lung cancer (with lung collapse)
	Uncommon
	Tuberculosis
	Exacerbation of bronchiectasis
	Idiopathic pulmonary fibrosis and other interstitial lung diseases
Non-respiratory causes	Cardiac
	Acute pulmonary oedema
	Acute myocardial infarction
	Bradyarrhythmia or tachyarrhythmia
	Aortic dissection
	Acute myocarditis
	Systemic disease
	Metabolic acidosis
	Severe anaemia
	Thyrotoxicosis
	Anxiety (hyperventilation)
	Severe sepsis
	Diabetic ketoacidosis

The physiological mechanisms behind the sensation of breathlessness are poorly understood. It is thought that the following mechanisms all play a part:

- resistance to the flow of air in and out of the lungs,
- abnormal sensations in stretch receptors in the respiratory muscles,
- increased sensation of the build-up of fluid at receptors in the lung substance and
- abnormal levels of carbon dioxide and oxygen in blood chemoreceptors.

History and clinical examination
In order to establish the cause of acute breathlessness, the clinical history is vital. However, if the patient is in acute respiratory

distress, emergency measures are often needed to stabilise the patient before a detailed history can be taken. In this case, the full examination and measurement of vital signs (blood pressure, heart and respiratory rate, oxygen saturations and temperature) are of paramount importance. Rapid assessment of the acutely ill patient, using the airway, breathing, circulation, disability and exposure (ABCDE) rule, and emergency measures such as high-flow oxygen and intravenous fluid save lives in this situation.

Ask the patient to describe how quickly the breathlessness started. Only two respiratory problems truly cause the 'sudden' onset of breathlessness: pneumothorax and pulmonary embolism (Chapman *et al.* 2009). Pneumothorax is common in two demographics: tall, thin, young males who are smokers and older adults with chronic obstructive pulmonary disease (COPD). Breathlessness is often accompanied by pleuritic chest pain (indeed some patients present with just chest pain). An acute pulmonary embolism is also a sudden event, and the patient will usually complain only of breathlessness, but it can be accompanied by pleuritic chest pain and haemoptysis.

A sudden onset of rapid palpitations may be accompanied by acute breathlessness in tachyarrhythmias such as ventricular tachycardia, supraventricular tachycardia or atrial fibrillation.

If the breathlessness has come on acutely, over minutes to hours, then pneumothorax and pulmonary embolism should still be considered as a diagnosis, but other causes become as likely. A patient with pneumonia will present with breathlessness of a few hours' duration unless the pneumonia is atypical, in which case the presentation may be over a few days. Fever, productive cough and systemic illness are usually present. If the patient has underlying airway disease such as asthma, bronchiectasis or COPD, then enquire about wheeze and symptoms suggesting infective exacerbations (fever or shivers, productive cough with purulent green sputum or, if the patient has chronic productive cough, a change in sputum colour, frequency or volume). A patient with pleural effusion usually presents with chronic breathlessness, but acute worsening and decompensation may occur, meaning that the patient attends the hospital as an emergency. The examination findings will

Table 2.2 Common causes of a pleural effusion.

Transudate (low protein content)	Exudate (high-protein content)
Heart failure	Lung cancer
Cirrhosis (chronic liver disease)	Pneumonia
Nephrotic syndrome of the kidney	Tuberculosis
Hypothyroidism	Bacterial pleural infection (empyema)
	Pulmonary embolism (infarction)
	Rheumatoid arthritis

usually make this clear. The causes of a pleural effusion are shown in Table 2.2.

Patients with endobronchial lung cancer are at risk of lobar or complete lung collapse when a tumour enlarges and completely obstructs an airway. Ask about features that suggest lung cancer – haemoptysis, chronic breathlessness, weight loss and persistent chest infection.

Cardiac causes must also be considered. Ask the patient about two features of breathlessness that relate to a cardiac cause: paroxysmal nocturnal dyspnoea, which describes waking up in the night, gasping for breath, and orthopnoea, which describes being unable to lie flat in bed. Indeed, ask the patient how many pillows they have to sleep with. Acute onset of breathlessness, with or without wheeze, may indicate heart failure (pulmonary oedema), and any pre-existing heart disease must be established, along with a history of angina pectoris.

Other than cardiorespiratory disease, there are a number of other common causes that should be considered. Ask the patient about blood loss and haematological disease (anaemia) and symptoms related to hypothyroidism (cold intolerance, weight gain, low mood, muscle pain and weakness). Also ask about a history of diabetes (diabetic ketoacidosis) and chronic kidney disease (metabolic acidosis). Breathlessness can only be reliably attributed to panic and anxiety (hyperventilation) if all other causes are ruled out. Indeed, it is dangerous to assume that because someone appears anxious, they may not have an underlying disease.

A good systemic clinical examination will reveal most causes of breathlessness. Focus on cardiac and respiratory examinations. Signs related to common respiratory diagnoses are shown in Table 2.3.

The onset of symptoms, associated features and any past medical history are important in making the diagnosis of acute breathlessness. Prompt examination and assessment of vital signs are key in establishing whether emergency measures are needed. Not all of the diagnoses will be clear after clinical assessment, and some basic tests will often be needed to seek subtler causes.

Specific investigations

Vital signs: blood pressure, respiratory rate, oxygen saturations, temperature and heart rate.

Peak expiratory flow (PEF): will be reduced in acute severe asthma.

Chest X-ray: will show consolidation in pneumonia, pneumothorax, chronic changes of COPD, pleural effusion and lung cancer and collapse. The chest X-ray is usually normal in pulmonary embolism.

Haemoglobin, thyroid function tests, urea and electrolytes: to look for non-respiratory causes.

White blood cell count, C-reactive protein (CRP) and blood cultures: to look for markers of infection.

Sputum culture: to isolate a causative organism if productive cough is present.

Arterial blood gas: to look for type 1 or 2 respiratory failure.

Computed tomography (CT) pulmonary angiogram: to look for pulmonary embolism.

Spiral CT of the thorax: to look for lung cancer and lobar or lung collapse.

Spirometry: to look for obstructive airway disease (COPD or asthma).

Echocardiogram: to look for signs of heart failure.

COUGH

Cough describes the rapid expulsion of exhaled material from the airways. Stimulation of the cough reflex results initially in

Table 2.3 Signs related to common respiratory diagnoses of acute breathlessness.

Cause	Signs on examination
Pulmonary embolism	High respiratory rate Normal chest expansion, percussion and auscultation Sinus tachycardia
Pneumonia	High respiratory rate Signs of consolidation (reduced chest expansion, reduced percussion note, bronchial breath sounds and coarse crackles on inspiration) Systemic inflammatory response (fever, sinus tachycardia, low blood pressure and poor capillary refill time)
Infective exacerbation of COPD	High respiratory rate, accessory muscle use and breathing with pursed lips Bilateral reduced chest expansion, global resonance to percussion and reduced breath sounds, with expiratory wheeze throughout Sinus tachycardia or irregular pulse (atrial fibrillation) Signs of pneumonia may also be present.
Acute severe asthma	High respiratory rate, accessory muscle use Bilateral reduced chest expansion, normal percussion and polyphonic expiratory wheeze throughout Sinus tachycardia Signs of pneumonia or viral infection may be present.
Pneumothorax	High respiratory rate Unilateral reduced chest expansion, hyper-resonance to percussion and absent breath sounds If the pneumothorax is under tension, there may be signs of respiratory distress, low blood pressure, collapse and deviation of the trachea away from the side of the lesion.
Massive pleural effusion	High respiratory rate Unilateral reduced chest expansion, stony dullness to percussion and reduced or absent breath sounds Tracheal deviation away from the side of the lesion
Lung collapse (usually secondary to lung cancer)	High respiratory rate Unilateral reduced chest expansion, dullness to percussion and bronchial breathing Tracheal deviation is towards the side of the lesion (because of volume loss).

closure of the glottis with a build-up of high expiratory pressures; the glottis is opened suddenly, and the contents are expelled. The medical name for cough is 'tussis', which is derived from the same Latin word (Martin 2010).

Cough is one of the most common presentations in primary care and also the most common symptom in respiratory disease (Kumar & Clark 2005). Smokers usually have a non-productive morning cough, while those with viral upper respiratory tract infections (for example a cold virus) and acute bronchitis have a cough often accompanied by other features of viral infection, such as fever, muscle and joint ache, headache, runny nose and sore throat. Other causes of cough need further evaluation. A cause for cough is not found in 10% of patients (Irwin & Madison 2000).

Cough is an important protective reflex mechanism that enables a normal patient to clear inhaled foreign body material from the lungs or remove excessive mucus secretions. The reflex is poorly understood, but cough receptors are present in the nose, larynx and upper and lower airways. Stimulation of these by irritants causes activation of afferent nerves which terminate in the cough centre of the medulla of the brain. A medullary reflex initiates a cough by activating the muscles of the upper airways and larynx. This cough reflex is diminished in patients with poor respiratory muscle function, such as those with neuromuscular disease, and patients taking opiate medication (Kumar & Clark 2005).

Causes
The causes of cough are shown in Table 2.4. It can be seen that most of the causes are related to respiratory disease, and diagnosis can be narrowed down by enquiring about other associated symptoms and particularly about the length of time the cough has been present.

History and clinical examination
The most important distinction is that of acute or chronic cough. Ask the patient about the duration of the cough. For example a chronic cough is defined as a cough with a duration of longer than 2 months (Irwin & Madison 2000).

Table 2.4   Causes of acute and chronic cough, listed with reference to important associated features.

	Associated features	**Causes**
Acute cough	Features of systemic infection, with or without sputum production	Upper respiratory tract infection – usually viral Acute bronchitis Whooping cough Infective exacerbation of COPD Pneumonia Tuberculosis
	Usually dry cough	Allergic rhinitis Lung cancer Acute exacerbation of asthma Acute smoke inhalation
Chronic cough (>2 months)	Dry cough	GORD Chronic asthma Interstitial lung disease Post-nasal drip Sinusitis Left ventricular failure Drugs such as ACE inhibitors
	Associated sputum production	Chronic bronchitis (COPD) Bronchiectasis Cystic fibrosis Recurrent aspiration pneumonia – in patients with stroke or neuromuscular disease

In acute cough, ask the patient about symptoms associated with infection, such as fever, sweats, muscle and joint ache, runny nose and sore throat. An acute cough productive of yellow or green sputum suggests viral or bacterial acute bronchitis. In pneumonia, the infection is usually severer; the patient may be breathless and have pleuritic chest pain or haemoptysis.

On examination, the presence of bronchial breathing and crackles differentiates bronchitis from pneumonia. Pneumonia is confirmed by consolidation on the chest X-ray. A paroxysmal 'whooping' cough which lasts for a number of weeks suggests infection with *Bordetella pertussis*, also known as whooping cough. This is usually an infection of childhood. Ask the patient about a previous history of COPD. Accompanying wheeze and acute breathlessness may indicate an exacerbation. A previous history of tuberculosis must be established, and features of active tuberculosis such as intermittent fevers and night sweats should be noted.

Ask about atopic features (eczema and hay fever) which may accompany allergic rhinitis, and enquire specifically about a runny or blocked nose, particularly in the summertime. Always enquire about smoking, as lung cancer can present in a number of ways, including recurrent infection or a cough, with or without haemoptysis.

Asthma has a number of features including chest tightness, wheeze and breathlessness but may present with only a chronic cough, which is worse at night or in the morning (diurnal variation). An acute exacerbation of asthma may occur in an asthma patient who does not normally cough. A history of asthma or accompanying wheeze and breathlessness may aid diagnosis.

A chronic cough lasts more than 2 months. The most important distinction to make is whether the cough is dry or productive of sputum. A chronic dry cough has a few common causes. Ask the patient about clinical features of gastro-oesophageal reflux disease (GORD). Ask specifically about acid reflux, indigestion and epigastric pain particularly after eating. Chronic asthma is another common cause, so ask about atopic features, respiratory symptoms in childhood and a family history of asthma. Establish associated features such as ongoing chest tightness, breathlessness, wheeze and diurnal variation. Ask about sinus infections and recurrent frontal headaches which may indicate chronic sinusitis. A post-nasal drip is usually produced at night when excessive mucus is produced by the sinuses and accumulates at the back of the throat, causing coughing, constant swallowing and clearing of the throat. It can be exacerbated by allergic rhinitis.

Progressive breathlessness and a dry cough with the presence of fine end-inspiratory crackles and clubbing on examination are likely to represent an interstitial lung disease. There are many of these diseases (more than 50!), and they used to be referred to under the umbrella term of 'lung fibrosis'. It is important to establish a history of exposure to allergens and irritants that cause interstitial lung disease. The common causes would be asbestos, coal dust, silica dust, moulds including *Aspergillus fumigatus*, pigeon and budgerigar antigen and occupation-related irritants such as isocyanate paint spray and metal dust. If any exposures are present, the patient is likely to need further investigations.

Ask specifically for a drug history, as treatment with angiotensin-converting enzyme (ACE) inhibitors can cause a dry cough which is not tolerated by the patient. The newer angiotensin-2 receptor blocker drugs have less incidence of chronic cough and are better tolerated.

A chronic cough with sputum production represents either the chronic bronchitis of COPD or chronic respiratory infection. In chronic bronchitis, the patient has a significant history of smoking (at least 20 cigarettes per day for 20 years) and initially coughs a small amount of clear or pale sputum (less than a tablespoon per day) for at least 3 months of the year. This is usually over the wintertime but can progress to all year round. The patient may be wheezy and breathless on exertion and may suffer with recurrent wheezy and infective exacerbations that require steroids and antibiotics.

Bronchiectasis is defined as irreversible bronchial dilation with chronic airway inflammation (Chapman *et al.* 2009). Sputum production is usually copious (more than an egg cup per day). The patient suffers frequent exacerbations requiring prolonged courses of antibiotics. The causes are shown in Table 2.5.

Table 2.5 Causes of bronchiectasis.

Post-infective causes	Tuberculosis Whooping cough Severe pneumonia
Genetic causes	Cystic fibrosis (pancreatic insufficiency)
Immune deficiency	Primary hypogammaglobulinaemia HIV infection Chronic leukaemias
Ciliary mucus clearance abnormalities	Primary ciliary dyskinesia Kartagener syndrome (situs inversus and sinusitis) Young syndrome (sinusitis and low sperm count)

Bronchiectasis can develop in a scarred lung after severe infection or can be part of a genetic disease, such as cystic fibrosis, or that of an immune deficiency. It is therefore important to ask about a family history of infection or genetic disease. However, it would be rare to see cystic fibrosis presenting for the first time in adulthood, because of the severe nature of the bronchiectasis in childhood.

Ask the patient about recent pneumonias, childhood infections and previous tuberculosis, and enquire specifically about infertility and sinusitis, which may suggest a rarer cause. Finally ask the patient about recurrent choking episodes, aspiration of food or drink and a previous history of stroke or neuromuscular disease. Bulbar nerve weakness can lead to poor swallowing and recurrent episodes of aspiration pneumonia.

Carry out a thorough clinical examination, paying particular attention to the respiratory system. Consolidation and crackles will be present in patients with pneumonia, to help differentiate it from acute bronchitis. A high respiratory rate and wheeze are usually present in acute asthma and infective exacerbations of COPD, with or without the presence of consolidation. A patient with weight loss, poor chest expansion bilaterally and accessory muscle use at rest may have chronic COPD rather than chronic asthma. Established weight loss may be evident in those with active tuberculosis and tar staining, cachexia, cervical lymphadenopathy and clubbing, and a pleural effusion may point towards a diagnosis of lung cancer. A patient with coarse inspiratory and expiratory crackles together with clubbing is likely to have bronchiectasis, whereas a patient with fine end-inspiratory crackles and clubbing is likely to have interstitial lung disease.

A cardiovascular examination may reveal signs of congestive or left ventricular failure, such as a laterally displaced apex beat, third heart sound, tachycardia and bibasal inspiratory crackles. Occasionally, severe heart failure may cause chronic cough alongside breathlessness. Examination of the nose and throat may reveal nasal and pharyngeal inflammation and cervical lymphadenopathy associated with upper respiratory tract infection. A runny nose, nasal polyps and watery eyes suggest allergic rhinitis. The patient may sneeze a lot. Chronic sinusitis may cause the patient's speech to become croaky or nasal, and

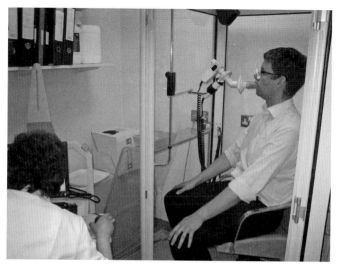

Figure 2.1   Full pulmonary function tests.

there may be tenderness over the frontal or maxillary sinuses (see Figure 2.1). Test the patient's swallowing by asking them to sip a teaspoon or a small glass of water. Choking or difficulty initiating swallowing suggests bulbar muscle weakness, and a cause for this should be sought, whether stroke disease or neuromuscular weakness.

Diseases causing respiratory muscle weakness are shown in Table 2.6. Measurement of vital signs is important. In acute cough, a high temperature, high respiratory rate, tachycardia, low blood pressure and low oxygen saturations may alert the clinician to features of serious systemic infection, and severe pneumonia or infective exacerbation of asthma or COPD is likely. In viral upper respiratory tract infection and acute bronchitis, the patient may have a fever but is unlikely to be systemically unwell, and these conditions are usually managed by the patient themselves or in the community.

The diagnosis of cough is broad and not necessarily related to local respiratory diseases. Classifying the cough by its duration and whether it is accompanied by sputum production are

Table 2.6 Diseases causing respiratory muscle weakness and poor cough reflex.

Systemic illness	Anaesthesia
	Coma
	Opiate and sedative drugs
	Severe COPD
Neuromuscular disease	Motor neurone disease
	Tetraplegia from spinal cord transection
	Duchene muscular dystrophy
	Myotonic dystrophy
Degenerative neurological disease	Stroke causing bulbar muscle dysfunction
	Bulbar palsy
	Parkinson's disease
	Guillain–Barre syndrome

the two most helpful measures in reasoning the diagnosis. The most prevalent cause of acute cough is viral upper respiratory tract infection. A chronic cough is commonly caused by GORD, a post-nasal drip or sinusitis, chronic asthma or drug therapy with ACE inhibitors. If a chronic cough persists, it requires more detailed investigation.

Specific investigations

Vital signs: blood pressure, respiratory rate, oxygen saturations, temperature and heart rate.

PEF: will be reduced in acute severe asthma. A PEF diary can be kept in chronic cough to look for chronic asthma and may show diurnal variation in PEF.

Chest X-ray: will show consolidation in pneumonia and tuberculosis. There may be hyperinflation in chronic asthma and COPD. A lung cancer may appear as a coin lesion or hilar enlargement, and there may be a pleural effusion. The chest X-ray can be normal in bronchiectasis, interstitial lung disease, chronic asthma and GORD. There may be chronic changes associated with heart failure.

White blood cell count, CRP and blood cultures: to look for markers of infection.

Sputum culture: to isolate a causative organism if productive cough is present.

Arterial blood gas: to look for type 1 or 2 respiratory failure, particularly in neuromuscular disease.

Spirometry, gas transfer and lung volumes (full pulmonary function tests; Figure 2.1): to look for COPD, chronic asthma (an obstructive pattern), interstitial lung disease (a restrictive pattern) or bronchiectasis (an obstructive or a restrictive pattern).

Reversibility testing or bronchial provocation testing: sometimes required to rule out or diagnose chronic asthma where the diagnosis is difficult.

High-resolution CT (HRCT) of the thorax: to look for characteristic changes of bronchiectasis or interstitial lung disease.

Spiral CT of the thorax: to look for lung cancer and lobar pneumonia.

Echocardiogram: to look for signs of heart failure.

Bronchoscopy (Figure 2.2): sometimes required in difficult cases, to exclude an endobronchial tumour, interstitial lung disease or tuberculosis. The cough reflex can also be assessed.

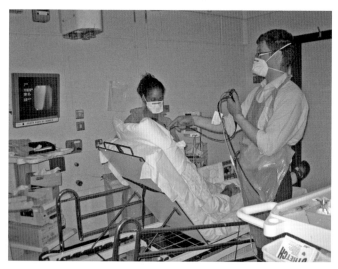

Figure 2.2 Bronchoscopy.

HAEMOPTYSIS

Haemoptysis describes the coughing up of blood (Martin 2010) from the lungs or airways. This should not be confused with haematemesis, which describes vomiting blood, that is, expulsion from the gastrointestinal tract. The blood may be in small amounts, in specks or streaks, or large amounts with clots and fresh blood. It may be accompanied by purulent sputum production. Haemoptysis is derived from the Greek words *haima* meaning blood and *ptysis*, which means spitting (Baert 2007).

Haemoptyis is a common and non-specific feature of many lung diseases, but it should always be taken seriously, as it may represent serious underlying pathology. In one third of cases, no cause is found (Chapman *et al*. 2009). Massive haemoptysis (up to 800 mL/24 h) is rare, but urgent opinion by a respiratory physician should be sought to prevent rapid deterioration in clinical condition.

Causes

The common causes of haemoptysis are few. The differential diagnosis usually lies between lung cancer, bronchiectasis, pulmonary embolism and tuberculosis (Chapman *et al*. 2009). Rarer causes exist, and these are all shown in Table 2.7.

Table 2.7 Common and rare causes of haemoptysis.

Common	Rare
Lung cancer (endobronchial tumour)	Vasculitis (for example Wegener's granulomatosis, systemic lupus erythematosus and Goodpasture's syndrome)
Pulmonary embolism	
Active tuberculosis	Arteriovenous malformation
Exacerbation of bronchiectasis	Hereditary haemorrhagic telangectasia
Severe pneumonia	Lung abscess
	Benign airway tumours
	Fungal infection
	Warfarin therapy
	Pulmonary haemosiderosis

History and clinical examination

Ask the patient if there is a past history of lung disease or haemoptysis; this may point straight towards the cause. Ask about the volume of blood; intermittent streaks or spots of blood would indicate small-volume haemoptysis, whereas multiple clots or egg-cup volumes would indicate large-volume haemoptysis. Ask about the time course. Constant and persistent haemoptysis is more likely to be due to lung cancer or a pulmonary embolism; intermittent haemoptysis is more likely to be active tuberculosis or recurrent infection in bronchiectasis.

Enquire about other symptoms of infection. Blood mixed with purulent sputum is more likely to represent the active infection of pneumonia, bronchiectasis or tuberculosis. However, lung cancer can cause bronchial obstruction and subsequent infection, so the patient should be asked about their smoking history and about persistent chest pain, weight loss and chronic cough. Enquire about risk factors for pulmonary embolism, such as immobility, presence of a deep-vein thrombosis, swollen leg, recent surgery, blood dyscrasias and a family history of thromboembolic disease.

Ensure that the blood is definitely being expelled from the airway rather than the nose, the mouth or the stomach. Haemoptysis can be mistaken for nosebleeds (epistaxis) or haematemesis. Occasionally, oral and pharyngeal infection and oral tumours can present with expulsion of blood from the mouth, so ask about difficulty swallowing (dysphagia) and oral pain and discharge. Take a drug history; the patient may be on warfarin or antiplatelet drugs which cause an increased risk of bleeding. However, there is still usually an underlying cause which promotes bleeding.

A general examination should be performed to look for signs associated with lung cancer: cachexia (extreme weight loss), clubbing, cervical lymphadenopathy or a Horner's syndrome. Pay careful attention to the respiratory examination. Respiratory distress may indicate a pulmonary embolism, pneumonia, an exacerbation of bronchiectasis or active tuberculosis. There may be signs of consolidation on chest examination that point towards pneumonia or tuberculosis. However, with a pulmonary embolism, lung cancer or some of the rarer causes such as arteriovenous malformation, the respiratory examination may be completely normal.

The diagnosis of haemoptysis can be straightforward if the patient has a history of lung disease which might promote bleeding. However, investigation with chest X-ray (and usually a CT modality scan) and bronchoscopy is nearly always required to conform the diagnosis. Rarer causes will only be picked up under direct vision at bronchoscopy, after a normal examination and chest X-ray. In one third of cases a bleeding point is never found, and the episode is isolated. However, persistent haemoptysis in a smoker suggests a more serious pathology and warrants urgent investigation.

Specific investigations

Vital signs: blood pressure, respiratory rate, oxygen saturations, temperature and heart rate. These may be altered, particularly in infection or tuberculosis.

Chest X-ray: will show consolidation in pneumonia and tuberculosis. A lung cancer may appear as a coin lesion or hilar enlargement, and there may be a pleural effusion. However, the chest X-ray can be normal in lung cancer, bronchiectasis and pulmonary embolism. Pulmonary infarction can occur from severe pulmonary embolism, and a wedge-shaped area of consolidation can appear.

White blood cell count, CRP and blood cultures: to look for markers of infection.

Sputum culture: to isolate a causative organism if productive cough is present.

Arterial blood gas: to look for type 1 respiratory failure in pneumonia and pulmonary embolism.

HRCT of the thorax: to look for characteristic changes of bronchiectasis or interstitial lung disease.

CT pulmonary angiogram: to look for pulmonary embolism.

Spiral CT of the thorax: to look for lung cancer, lobar consolidation, active tuberculosis, lung abscesses and vasculitic areas of haemorrhage.

Bronchoscopy: usually required to exclude an endobronchial tumour or to take washings to look for active tuberculosis or fungal infection. Rarer causes, namely arteriovenous malformations, rare benign tumours of the upper airways, haemorrhagic telangectasia and lung abscesses, can also be seen.

DIGITAL CLUBBING

Digital clubbing (Figure 2.3) describes enlargement of the terminal segments of the fingers and/or toes, which results from overgrowth of connective tissue between the nail and the distal phalanx (Myers & Farquhar 2001). It is usually symmetrical, affecting all fingers (or toes), but can occur on one hand (or one foot) only. It was first described by Hippocrates over 2000 years ago, and the name relates to the drumstick shape of the fingers in severe disease.

Clubbing can be hereditary or idiopathic, but more often it is a sign of underlying disease (Karnath 2003). It is common in suppurative lung diseases, lung malignancy and cyanotic congenital heart disease. Clubbing is present in up to a third of

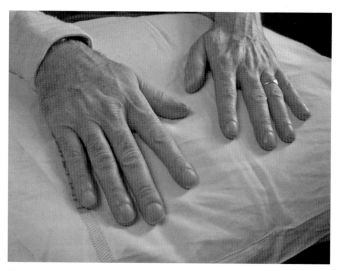

Figure 2.3 Digital clubbing.

Table 2.8   Causes of digital clubbing.

Malignant respiratory disease	Malignant disease
	    Bronchial carcinoma
	    Mesothelioma
	Suppurative disease
	    Lung abscess
	    Bronchiectasis
	    Cystic fibrosis
	    Empyema
	Interstitial lung disease

Cardiovascular	Cyanotic congenital heart disease Infective endocarditis
Gastrointestinal	Liver cirrhosis Crohn's disease Ulcerative colitis Coeliac disease
Metabolic disease	Hypothyroidism
Hereditary	Autosomal dominant inheritance
Idiopathic digital clubbing	

patients presenting with lung cancer (Sridhar *et al.* 1998) and is more common in non–small-cell lung cancer.

Causes

Clubbing is associated with a variety of diseases which are all subacute or chronic in nature. These diseases are infectious, neoplastic, inflammatory or vascular. The most common causes are respiratory or cardiovascular in origin. The causes of clubbing are shown in Table 2.8.

Nail bed thickness is usually less than 2 mm. Clubbed fingers show an increased nail bed thickness and low density of normal nail bed connective tissue. There is a proliferation of growth and inflammatory cells (fibroblasts, eosinophils and lymphocytes) and also of small blood vessels. There is no consensus as to the mechanism behind it, particularly in those with hereditary or idiopathic clubbing.

It is thought that growth is stimulated by low tissue oxygen levels, particularly in those with respiratory and cyanotic heart disease; however, this does not explain the pathophysiology in other diseases. In lung cancer, clubbing is associated with hypertrophic osteoarthropathy which is a condition that causes swelling of bone lining (periosteum) and painful bone and joint extremities. Because of its association with cancer, it is called a 'paraneoplastic' phenomenon.

History and clinical examination

It is important to exclude all serious causes of clubbing before attributing the condition to being hereditary or idiopathic. Ask the patient whether they have had the condition since childhood (which makes the hereditary cause, congenital heart disease and cystic fibrosis likely) or whether it has had a recent onset (which makes the other causes more likely). Enquire about a family history of clubbing, but appreciate that diseases such as cystic fibrosis also have a genetic component to them.

Ask about common respiratory symptoms – breathlessness, wheeze, chest pain and cough with or without sputum production. Associated respiratory symptoms make a respiratory cause more likely. Be sure to ask about haemoptysis, weight loss, sweats, fevers and features of systemic infection. These will point you towards a suppurative or malignant cause. Clubbing with an onset in middle age with a dry cough and breathlessness is more likely to be due to idiopathic pulmonary fibrosis, which is a very common cause.

Ask the patient about bowel symptoms – pale fatty stools, abdominal colicky pains, diarrhoea and intolerance of wheat all suggest celiac disease. Intermittent diarrhoea with or without blood in the stool, with cramping lower abdominal pains, suggests inflammatory bowel disease. Jaundice, right upper quadrant pain and a history of high alcohol intake or previously diagnosed hepatitis suggest cirrhosis of the liver. It can be seen that many of these causes can be differentiated by a good history.

A patient with congenital heart disease will usually have a previous history of paediatric cardiac surgery or at least a knowledge of previous consultations. Enquire about the symptoms associated with hypothyroidism – weight gain, intolerance of cold, palpitations, fatigue, increased daytime sleepiness, croaky voice and low mood.

Clinical examination should concentrate on the respiratory and cardiovascular system, looking for signs associated with malignant, suppurative or inflammatory disease, not forgetting to undertake a brief examination of thyroid function, looking for signs of hypothyroidism – a goitre, slow reflexes, bradycardia, obesity and proximal muscle weakness.

Although clubbing can be a benign or hereditary condition, the implications in an adult are such that its detection on examination should prompt further questioning and investigation to look for an underlying cause. In those who are asymptomatic, a chest X-ray should be performed at the very least, particularly if the patient is a smoker.

Specific investigations

Vital signs: blood pressure, respiratory rate, oxygen saturations, temperature and heart rate. These may be altered, particularly in chronic infection.

Chest X-ray: will show consolidation and cavitation in infections or exacerbations of bronchiectasis. A lung cancer may appear as a coin lesion or hilar enlargement. Pleural effusion may be present and may indicate an empyema.

White blood cell count, CRP and blood cultures: to look for markers of infection and inflammation.

Thyroid function tests, coeliac antibodies and liver function tests: to look for non-respiratory causes.

Sputum culture: to isolate a causative organism if productive cough is present.

Sodium or chloride sweat test: to look for cystic fibrosis.

12-lead electrocardiogram and echocardiogram: to look for cyanotic heart disease.

Liver ultrasound scan: to look for cirrhosis of the liver.

HRCT of the thorax: to look for characteristic changes of bronchiectasis (including cystic fibrosis) or interstitial lung disease.

Spiral CT of the thorax: to look for lung cancer, lung abscesses and cavitating infection. The pleural space may contain pus or thickened walls, which indicates empyema.

Bronchoscopy: may be required to exclude an endobronchial tumour or to take washings to look for active infection or an abscess.

INSPIRATORY STRIDOR

Stridor is the noise heard on breathing when the larynx or the trachea is obstructed (Martin 2010). It tends to be louder and harsher than expiratory wheeze and is often more obvious during inspiration, when it is heard as a distinctive crowing or snoring noise. Upper airway obstruction is a life-threatening emergency, and prompt identification and management is essential.

Patients with upper airway obstruction are seen frequently in emergency departments, and all staff should be trained in the emergency management of acute upper airway obstruction. Common cases involve airway burns and smoke inhalation, anaphylaxis, laryngeal infection and foreign body aspiration. Upper airway obstruction is also seen in inpatients, particularly those who are critically ill and those with existing neck and mediastinal disease, and also in perioperative patients.

Causes

The causes of inspiratory stridor are shown in Table 2.9. Broadly, the obstruction can be within the upper airway (the lumen of the

Table 2.9 Causes of inspiratory stridor.

Intrathoracic obstruction	Pharyngeal occlusion by tongue (because of coma, drugs, alcohol and stroke)
	Anaphylaxis
	Oedema from burns (smoke inhalation)
	Foreign body in larynx or trachea (also causes laryngeal spasm)
	Aspiration of blood or vomit
	Epiglottitis or laryngitis
	Vocal cord dysfunction
	Laryngeal tumour
Extrathoracic obstruction	Goitre
	Thyroid haemorrhage (usually post-surgical)
	Lymphadenopathy

larynx or trachea), because of swelling of the wall of the upper airway or from external compression.

History and clinical examination

Stridor is a symptom rather than a diagnosis, and it is important to find the underlying cause. Stridor is a loud, harsh and high-pitched noise. It can start as a low-pitched 'croaking' and, when severer, progresses to a high-pitched 'crowing'. It is usually heard only on inspiration because of partial collapsibility and obstruction of the airway. Being heard on inspiration and expiration usually indicates either severe upper airway obstruction or large bronchus obstruction.

The initial management should follow the ABCDE rule, concentrating on securing the airway and enabling adequate oxygenation. Subsequent management will depend upon the underlying diagnosis. Senior anaesthetic help and advice from senior staff should be sought immediately after basic emergency measures taken. In a patient who has experienced complete obstruction and has become unconscious, emergency measures to secure the airway with an endotracheal tube will need to be taken. If the obstruction is due to foreign body matter, a Heimlich manoeuvre should be performed to attempt to dislodge the obstruction.

If the patient presents to the accident and emergency department, it is important to establish the history of the preceding minutes or hours. This may come from the patient or a family member or friend if the patient is too unwell. Smoke inhalation and foreign body inhalation are usually clear immediately from the history. You will need to enquire further about vomiting, preceding respiratory tract infection causing laryngitis and epiglottitis, history of laryngeal or bronchial tumour or any known allergens. Vocal cord dysfunction occurs in the presence of chronic and often-unstable asthma, and previous episodes are common.

Clinical examination may reveal features of anaphylaxis – low blood pressure, tachycardia, facial or neck swelling, an urticarial rash and wheeze on the chest. Extrathoracic compression from a thyroid mass or neck lymph node enlargement may be obvious from a past medical history of thyroid or malignant disease, but a goitre or lymph node mass may be palpable.

Prompt recognition of upper airway obstruction allows early emergency management strategies to prevent complete airway obstruction and cardiovascular collapse. The history will reveal the cause in many cases, but this should not delay following the ABCDE of resuscitation!

Specific investigations

The cause of upper airway obstruction may not be obvious on clinical encounter, and early anaesthetic and ENT input may allow urgent visualisation of the upper airway by *laryngoscopy* and insertion of an *endotracheal tube* by the anaesthetists or by *fibre-optic endoscopy* on the part of the ENT surgeons, depending on the urgency and which is more appropriate. A *chest X-ray* may reveal a superior mediastinal mass which is compressing the trachea. Sometimes a *soft-tissue cervical X-ray* will reveal a foreign body obstruction.

REFERENCES

Baert, A.L. (ed.) (2007) *Encyclopaedia of Diagnostic Imaging*. Springer, Philadelphia.

Chapman, S., Robinson, G., Stradling, J.R.S., *et al.* (2009) *The Oxford Handbook of Respiratory Medicine*, 2nd edn. Oxford University Press, Oxford.

Cox, N. & Roper, T. (2005) *Clinical Skills: Oxford Core Text*. Oxford University Press, Oxford.

Irwin, R.S. & Madison, J.M. (2000) The diagnosis and treatment of cough. *New England Journal of Medicine* **343**, 1715–1721.

Karnath, B. (2003) Digital clubbing: a sign of underlying disease. *Hospital Physician* **26**, 25–27.

Kumar, P. & Clark, M. (2005) *Clinical Medicine*, 6th edn. W.B. Saunders, Edinburgh, UK.

Marcovitch, H. (2005) *Black's Medical Dictionary*. 41st edn. A & C Black, London.

Martin, A. (ed.) (2010) *Oxford Concise Medical Dictionary*, 8th edn. Oxford University Press, Oxford.

Myers, K.A. & Farquhar, D.R. (2001) The rational clinical examination. Does this patient have clubbing? *Journal of the American Medical Association* **286** (3), 341–347.

Sridhar, K.S., Lobo, C.F. & Altman, R.D. (1998) Digital clubbing and lung cancer. *Chest* **114**, 1535–1537.

3 | Clinical Diagnosis of Symptoms Associated with the Cardiovascular System

Yonas Mhando and Phil Jevon

The aim of this chapter is to understand the clinical diagnosis of symptoms associated with the cardiovascular system.

LEARNING OUTCOMES
At the end of this chapter, the reader will be able to discuss the clinical diagnosis of the following symptoms associated with the cardiovascular system:

❑ chest pain,
❑ palpitations,
❑ hypertension,
❑ calf swelling,
❑ bruising,
❑ leg ulcer and
❑ anaemia,
❑ Hypotension.

CHEST PAIN
Chest pain is a symptom of a number of medical conditions ranging from trivial to life-threatening. Usually considered as a medical emergency, it is one of most common reasons for patients to seek medical advice. Although acute coronary syndrome (ACS) is the most common cause of chest pain, there

Clinical Diagnosis, 1st edition. Edited by Phil Jevon.
© 2011 Blackwell Publishing Ltd.

are many other causes, some life-threatening and some trivial (Raftery *et al.* 2010). It is therefore essential to have knowledge of various causes of chest pain as well as being able to assess and describe the patients' condition and assist in determining the correct diagnosis so that effective clinical management can be instituted without undue delay.

Causes

The most common cause of chest pain is ACS. This term encompasses two main conditions, namely acute myocardial infarction (AMI) and unstable angina (UA). Both conditions require urgent assessment and investigation to confirm diagnosis. Stable angina pectoris which is not part of ACS is defined as pain resulting from inadequate blood supply to the myocardium.

Unstable angina

It is described as recurrent episodes of angina occurring on minimal exertion or at rest. It is termed 'crescendo angina' when it occurs with increasing frequency over a few days and is progressively provoked by less exertion. Unstable angina can also present with prolonged pain similar to that of AMI but without the electrocardiogram (ECG) and cardiac enzyme changes consistent with AMI. In most cases, unstable angina represents deterioration of a previously stable angina, but it can also represent initial presentation of ischaemic heart disease (IHD).

Pain is often associated with reversible ST depression on the ECG, but the ECG can be normal or show non-specific abnormalities.

Myocardial infarction

Myocardial infarction (MI) can be either non-Q-wave or Q-wave MI. In both conditions, the patient usually presents with clinical features of ACS, and cardiac enzyme levels are significantly elevated to indicate myocardial damage. However, in non-Q-wave MI, ECG changes are non-specific (ST-depression, T-wave inversion), whereas in Q-wave MI, ECG shows ST elevation, and Q waves eventually develop in the leads that display ST elevation (Jevon 2009).

Other common causes of chest pain include the following (Jevon *et al*. 2008, Llewelyn *et al*. 2009, Raftery *et al*. 2010):

Pulmonary embolism: sudden or subacute onset chest pain occurring in relation to pulmonary infarction and often described as pleuritic in nature (sharp and worsening with inspiration). It is usually associated with breathlessness, haemoptysis or collapse. Patients must be assessed and treated urgently.

Pericarditis: usually sharp pain exacerbated by inspiration and relieved by sitting forward. It is due to inflammation of the pericardium and is commonly associated with pyrexia and responds well to non-steroidal anti-inflammatory drugs. Auscultation of the chest may reveal pericardial rub.

Pneumothorax: sudden-onset pain localised on the affected side of the chest. Patients have usually breathless, and the severity of breathlessness is proportional to the size and type of pneumothorax. Risk factors for pneumothorax include chronic obstructive pulmonary disease (COPD), chest trauma, previous pneumothorax and being a tall and thin young individual. A chest X-ray can confirm the diagnosis.

Dissecting aortic aneurysm: sudden onset pain, usually described as 'tearing' or 'ripping' and commonly radiates to the back or the shoulder blades. This is an emergency.

Pneumonia: usually pleuritic-type chest pain associated with productive cough, fever and breathlessness.

Pleurisy: this is associated with inflammation of the pleura which commonly occurs in viral chest infection, pneumonia and pulmonary infarction secondary to pulmonary embolism.

Problems associated with the chest wall: any injury to the chest wall, costochondritis (a benign and harmless condition but often mistaken for cardiac pain), shingles and spinal nerve pain.

Gastro-oesophageal reflux disease: the pain can mimic cardiac pain in that it can radiate to the jaw and the throat, and it is often mistaken for cardiac pain.

History and clinical examination
A prompt history, clinical examination and initial investigations are paramount in patients presenting with chest pain because it could indicate a life-threatening illness. The airway, breathing, circulation, disability and exposure (ABCDE) approach of the

Resuscitation Council UK (2006) to the assessment of the critically ill patient is paramount (see Chapter 2).

The importance of history taking in respect of any pain has been discussed in Chapter 2.

In particular, the following should be noted:

Character: for example, central crushing chest pain, like a tight vice around the chest, is usually cardiac in origin. Chest pain may be absent in elderly and diabetic patients. In such cases, presenting symptoms may include collapse, epigastric pain, dyspnoea and acute confusional state. Chest pain worse on inspiration may indicate illness such as pleurisy or pericarditis. A 'tearing' or 'ripping' chest pain radiating to the back or the shoulder blades may be due to a dissecting aortic aneurysm.

Location: for example, retrosternal chest pain radiating to the left arm, jaw and neck usually indicates a cardiac origin but may also be caused by oesophageal reflux (Raftery *et al*. 2010).

Precipitating and relieving factors: for example, chest pain precipitated by exercise but relieved by rest suggests angina.

Note any risk factors for IHD:

modifiable risk factors, for example smoking, hypertension, hypercholestrolaemia, obesity, diabetes mellitus, sedentary lifestyle and stress;

non-modifiable risk factors, for example age, male sex, family history of premature MI in a first-degree relative (<55 years of age) and premature menopause.

Specific investigations

12-lead ECG: evidence of ACS (Figure 3.1).

Chest X-ray.

Cardiac enzymes and troponin levels.

Coronary angiography.

VQ scan: if pulmonary embolism suspected.

PALPITATIONS

'Palpitations' is the term used to describe the abnormal awareness of the heartbeats. Occasional awareness of one's own heartbeats can be normal, but when it occurs frequently, it can

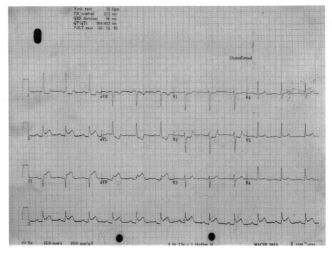

Figure 3.1 Acute coronary syndrome.

indicate that the underlying pathological conditions usually are of cardiac or metabolic origin or are drug induced. Episodes of palpitations can last for a few seconds or occasionally for hours. Investigations are always necessary when palpitations are associated with other symptoms such as sweating, chest pain, dizziness and syncope.

Causes

Generally, causes of palpitations can be categorized into three main groups:

- Hyperdynamic circulation: for example in valvular incompetence, thyrotoxicosis, hypercapnia, pyrexia, severe anaemia and pregnancy.
- Sympathetic overdrive: for example panic attacks, adrenaline, hypoglycaemia, antihystamines, alcohol, caffeine, heart failure and valvular heart disease such as mitral stenosis.
- Cardiac arrhythmias: for example atrial fibrillation, supraventricular tachycardia, ventricular tachycardia, ventricular fibrillation and heart blocks.

History and clinical examination

The most valuable initial clues to the diagnosis are the history and the description of the palpitations. It is important to establish whether there is any precipitating factor and how palpitations start and stop, as well as the approximate pulse rate during the attack. Alcohol, caffeine and illicit drug (such as cocaine and amphetamines) consumption should be enquired in the history as well as past history of IHD, anaemia, hypertension, hyperthyroidisms, panic attacks, stress and anxiety.

Irregular fast palpitations are most likely to be due to paroxysmal atrial fibrillation or atrial flutter with variable atrioventricular block. Regular fast palpitations are likely to be due to supraventricular tachycardia or anxiety. Atrial and ventricular ectopics are usually associated with awareness of missed or dropped beats. If palpitations are slow, the underlying cause is likely to be bigeminus or drugs such as beta-blockers and calcium channel blockers.

Often the cause of palpitations is unknown, but sometimes it can be precipitated by exercise, excessive tea or coffee intake, alcohol and illicit drug use, for example the use of cocaine and amphetamines. Anaemia and anxiety can worsen palpitations.

Symptoms of palpitation may often be just the feeling of an abnormal heartbeat. Palpitations do not always suggest the presence of cardiac disease, but this diagnosis is likely and should always be considered, if palpitations are associated with one or more of the following:

- chest tightness or pain,
- breathlessness,
- dizziness,
- sweating and
- syncope.

For any type of palpitation, the assessing clinician should establish the heart rate clinically and by an ECG. The clinician should treat the patient and not the heart rate. The most important task is to establish whether the patient is compromised by palpitations or not.

Physical examination and ECG are crucial in the assessment of palpitations, but often they do not uncover the diagnosis, as the patient may be asymptomatic at the time of assessment. Examination can be completely normal or can give clues such as irregular pulse, heart murmur, clinical signs of anaemia, heart failure, sepsis or thyroid disease.

Specific investigations

12-lead ECG: should be recorded preferably during an episode of palpitations. In an acute setting, a patient with recurrent or continuous palpitation requires cardiac monitoring to increase the chance of identifying the underlying rhythm abnormalities and help monitoring therapy if the patient is already on treatment.

24-hour ECG tape: continuous ambulatory cardiac monitoring usually for a period of 24-hour, but monitoring can be longer (up to 48-hour or more) if palpitations occur infrequently.

Continuous-loop recorder: a 'patient-activated recorder' can be helpful when palpitations are infrequent in people with very infrequent, but disabling, symptoms.

Thyroid function test: to exclude hyperthyroid disease as the possible cause of palpitations.

Renal function, serum magnesium and calcium levels: essential in assessing electrolytes and metabolic abnormalities.

Echocardiogram: to identify any structural heat disease or presence of intracardiac thrombus, especially when palpitations are due to atrial fibrillation.

HYPERTENSION

It is very difficult to define hypertension, and indeed there is no single blood pressure (BP) value above which hypertension can be defined definitively, but it is currently generally acceptable to consider treating BP above 140/90 mmHg as high, especially in presence of other risk factors for IHD and cerebrovascular disease. BP rises with age, and this rise is more noticeable in systolic pressure. Equally, mortality and morbidity risk increases with rising systolic and diastolic pressures. In any population, BP is distributed around a mean level, and more people have high BP than low. It is therefore imperative to have an individualized approach in diagnosing and treating hypertension.

Hypertension is a major but preventable risk factor for IHD. It affects approximately one third to half of the population in Western countries. The condition remains largely asymptomatic until complications due to end-organ damage occur; hence, it is often referred to as the 'silent killer'.

Causes

Hypertension can be classified into three main categories (Beevers *et al*. 2007, British Hypertensive Society 2010).

Primary hypertension

Primary hypertension (also known as essential or idiopathic hypertension) accounts for over 90% of all cases of hypertension. Some individuals (usually younger than 50 years) have the so-called classical essential hypertension which is defined as raised diastolic and/or systolic BP. Isolated systolic hypertension (systolic pressure $\geq$ 160/diastolic pressure $<$ 90 mmHg) is more common in older individuals. General causes include the following:

- multifactorial factors, namely genetic, familial and environmental factors;
- environmental factors, namely heavy alcohol consumption, high salt intake and stress;
- obesity;
- race and sex.

Secondary hypertension

An individual is said to have secondary hypertension when a specific cause has been found. This diagnosis should be strongly considered in those presenting with hypertension at a young age. This is especially important because this type of hypertension can often be cured completely. A number of causes have been identified, including the following:

- Renal diseases account for 80% of all cases of secondary hypertension. Common causes are renal artery stenosis, diabetic nephropathy, chronic interstitial renal disease and polycystic kidney disease.
- Endocrine diseases, namely Cushing disease, Conn's syndromes, adrenal hyperplasia and phaeochromocytoma, also cause hypertension.
- Pregnancy – hypertension detected in the second half of pregnancy usually resolves after delivery. If detected in the first half of pregnancy, it is probably due to pre-existing essential hypertension.
- Coarctation of the aorta is an important cardiovascular cause of hypertension.

White coat hypertension

Individuals are said to have 'white coat hypertension' if they exhibit significantly elevated BP in a clinical setting but a normal level when recording their own BP at home. The term is derived from the fact that traditionally doctors tend to wear white coats. The main cause of white coat hypertension is believed to be the fear and anxiety experienced by individuals in a clinic visit and during consultation.

Ambulatory BP monitoring and patient self-recording using a home BP recording device can be used to differentiate white coat hypertension from true chronic hypertension.

History and clinical examination

Except for malignant hypertension, hypertension is an asymptomatic condition and can therefore present late with end-organ complications. Sweating and palpitations may suggest phaeochromocytoma, while breathlessness may indicate the presence of left ventricular hypertrophy and heart failure.

The history should establish patient's age, sex and ethnic background. Ask about family history of hypertension, IHD, kidney disease, diabetes and dyslipidaemia. Enquire about stress, lifestyle, alcohol consumption and smoking. Steroids, oral contraceptive pills and vasopressin may all cause hypertension, and the use of these drugs should be specifically enquired in the history. If appropriate, the history should not be concluded without enquiry about pregnancy.

Obesity, sedentary lifestyle, stress, cigarette smoking and excessive alcohol consumption are all known to worsen hypertension or make it less responsive to treatment.

Mild hypertension is usually asymptomatic. Episodic sweating and palpitations may indicate secondary hypertension usually because of phaeochromocytoma. In severe hypertension, especially when complications have occurred, the following symptoms may be present:

- headaches;
- epistaxis;
- dyspnoea;
- symptoms of heart failure;
- seizure, for example in malignant hypertension;
- visual disturbances due to hypertensive retinopathy;
- abdominal mass palpable (polycystic kidney, phaeochromocytoma) or audible bruit of renal artery stenosis and
- presence of diminished femoral artery pulsations in coarctation of the aorta.

Usually, the only evident abnormality is the elevated BP. One should check for

- renal artery bruit which may be present in renavascular hypertension;
- radio-femoral pulse delay in coarctation of the aorta;
- clinical evidence of left ventricular hypertrophy and heart failure (for example third heart sound) and
- hypertensive retinopathy.

Specific investigations

12-lead ECG: may show evidence of left ventricular hypertrophy or coronary heart disease.

Chest radiography: may show cardiomegaly or pulmonary oedema if significant left ventricular heart failure is present.

Rib notching may suggest coarctation of the aorta as the cause of hypertension.

Urinalysis: significant proteinuria can be an indicator of renal complication due to long standing hypertension or the presence of primary renal disease causing hypertension.

Fasting glucose and lipid profile: diabetes may be diagnosed.

Renal function test and estimated glomerular filtration rate: if creatinine is raised, further renal workup investigations should be carried out. Low potassium suggests a diagnosis of Cushing disease or hyperaldosteronism.

Echocardiography: may be necessary to confirm left ventricular hypertrophy and the presence and severity of heart failure.

CALF SWELLING

The calf is said to be swollen when there is noticeable increase in its circumference. In most cases, the swelling is due to oedema. One or more specific conditions may be responsible for formation of oedema. Calf swelling is more prevalent in adults than in paediatric population.

Causes

Causes of unilateral calf swelling include the following:

- deep-venous thrombosis (DVT),
- cellulitis,
- ruptured Baker's cyst,
- chronic venous insufficiency,
- thrombophlebitis,
- compartment syndrome and
- acute lower limb ischaemia.

Causes of bilateral swelling include the following:

- peripheral oedema due to heart failure, hypoalbuminaemia or nephrotic syndrome;
- bilateral chronic venous insufficiency and
- lymphoedema.

History and clinical examination

A careful history should be taken with a view to establishing the nature and duration of swelling, as well as risk factors for various causes of calf swelling. Acute or subacute unilateral calf pain with redness, swelling and fever are typical features of cellulitis. DVT is more likely if there is unilateral calf swelling and pain but no fever. A ruptured Baker's cyst or knee joint should be suspected if the onset of swelling is sudden, if there is history of rheumatoid arthritis and if there is bruising or knee effusion. Also, the following should be enquired in history:

- onset and duration of swelling;
- any recent leg trauma or recent operation;
- previous calf swelling;
- history immobility or malignancy;
- past history of heart failure, pulmonary embolism, DVT, varicose veins and diabetes;
- pregnancy and recent child delivery, long-haul flights and use of oral contraceptive pills;
- risk factors for peripheral vascular disease, for example atrial fibrillation, hypertension, hypercholesteronaemia and smoking;
- chest pain or breathlessness.

Some causes of calf swelling are serious, while others are benign. In most cases diagnosis is usually easy to make, but DVT is easy to miss, especially in the post-operative period where it may be present without any physical sign. Diagnosis of DVT requires a high degree of clinical suspicion. Diagnosis and management of DVT can be straightforward in elderly and male patients but require important considerations in young female patients and in pregnancy, as it will influence contraceptive advice and delivery arrangement in the respective cases.

- Inspect the calves for size and symmetry, swelling, bruises, rashes, discoloration, ulcer and bulging of leg veins (present in superficial thrombophlebitis).
- Feel the calves for temperature (compare both sides).
- Check for tenderness.
- Check for oedema – pitting sign.

> **Box 3.1   Wells score (possible score −2 to 9)**
>
> - Active cancer (treatment within last 6 months or palliative) – 1 point
> - Calf swelling >3 cm compared with the other calf (measured 10 cm below tibial tuberosity) – 1 point
> - Collateral superficial veins (non-varicose) – 1 point
> - Pitting oedema (confined to the symptomatic leg) – 1 point
> - Swelling of the entire leg – 1 point
> - Localized pain along the distribution of the deep venous system – 1 point
> - Paralysis, paresis or recent cast immobilization of lower extremities – 1 point
> - Recently bedridden for more than 3 days or major surgery requiring regional or general anaesthetic in the past 4 weeks – 1 point
> - Alternative diagnosis at least as likely – subtract 2 points
>
> Score of 2 or higher: DVT is likely. Consider imaging the leg veins.
> Score of less than 2: DVT is unlikely. Consider blood test such as the D-dimer test to further rule out DVT.

- Examine for signs of acute ischaemia – pallor, cold, pain, paraesthesia, pulselessness and paralysis.
- Carry out Homans's test: dorsiflexion of the foot elicits pain in the posterior calf (suggestive of DVT).
- Look for Pratt's sign: squeezing of the posterior calf elicits pain (suggestive of DVT).

Assessment should include DVT probability scoring using Wells score (Box 3.1), which is a set of clinical prediction rules for the presence or absence of DVT.

Specific investigations

D-dimer: a useful and relevant test if DVT is suspected. An elevated D-dimer result suggests DVT as the cause of calf swelling. A low D-dimer level in a patient with low clinical probability of DVT should prompt alternative diagnoses, for example a ruptured Baker's cyst.

Doppler ultrasound scan (Figure 3.1): can be used to confirm or exclude DVT when D-dimer is elevated. It is also useful in assessing other causes of calf swelling, for example a ruptured Baker's cyst and arterial disease.

Clotting studies: to look for coagulopathy.

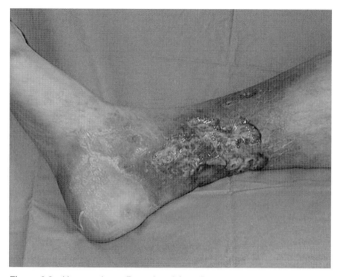

Figure 3.2 Venous ulcers. Reproduced from Donnelly & London (2009), with permission from John Wiley and Sons.

LEG ULCER

An ulcer refers to tissue breakdown due to any cause. In a leg ulcer the skin and underlying tissues are usually affected.

Leg ulcers are common in developed countries. The cause of leg ulcers can often be identified from a combination of the history, examination findings, the site of the ulcer and the patient's circumstances.

Venous ulcers (Figure 3.2) are by far the most common type of leg ulcers, and their incidence is more marked in the developing world. They often occur as a result of persistent venous hypertension and are more common in the elderly population (Gohel & Poskitt 2009). The common site for these types of ulcers is in the lower leg, just above the ankle. Venous ulcers can be associated with varicose veins, venous eczema, pigmentations, scarring atrophy, telangiectasia and DVT. Severe pain is a common symptom in venous ulcers and is more pronounced when there is associated infection.

Arterial ulcers are usually seen higher up on the leg or on the foot. They are usually painful and have a 'punch-out' appearance. Patients with arterial ulcers will almost always have symptoms and risk factors for peripheral vascular disease and coronary artery disease such as hypertension, angina, intermittent claudication, distal leg pain when supine and smoking history. Examination of the leg may show atrophic skin changes, pallor, cold cyanotic foot or toes, diminished or absent peripheral pulses, arterial bruits and absence of bleeding in the ulcer. The foot becomes pale on elevation, and redness occurs on lowering the foot.

Neuropathic ulcers occur as a result of repeated trauma over the pressure areas of the feet in patients with reduced sensation in the feet due to polyneuropathy. The common site is at the head of the metatarsal on the plantar aspect of the feet, and the ulcers are typically painless. They are commonly seen in patients with diabetes or leprosy.

Causes

Causes of leg ulcers include the following (Donnelly & London 2009, Raftery *et al*. 2010):

- venous insufficiency;
- arterial insufficiency;
- neuropathic ulcer (associated with diabetes and leprosy);
- haematological conditions such as sickle cell disease and spherocytosis;
- malignancy such as melanoma and squamous and basal cell carcinoma;
- infection, for example syphilis, tuberculosis, fungal infection and yaws;
- vasculitis, for example rheumatoid arthritis, pyoderma gangrenosum and systemic lupus erythematosus;
- pyoderma gangrenosum associated with inflammatory bowel disease, rheumatoid arthritis and myeloproliferative disorders;
- varicose veins;
- ischaemic arterial ulceration, usually in the anterior or lateral lower leg and cold pulseless cyanotic foot;

- vasculitis associated with rheumatoid arthritis and other connective tissue diseases and
- sustained pressure over joint or bone prominence, for example pressure sore.

History and clinical examination

A detailed history should be undertaken to identify any of the above-mentioned possible causes of the leg ulcer. Clinical examination should include close inspection of the leg for evidence of poor circulation, for example pallor, cool peripheries and weak pulses. The ulcer itself should be closely examined.

Specific investigations

Dopplar ultrasound scan.
Arteriography and venography: to assess circulation.
Biopsy: if carcinoma is suspected.
Blood glucose and cholesterol: to assess risk factors for peripheral vascular disease.

BRUISING

A bruise or an ecchymosis is a large bleeding into the skin. A small circumscribed bleeding into the skin is known as a purpura. Increasing age is associated with the likelihood of bruising. Bruises are usually painless, but occasionally pain may be present, especially when bruises are associated with injury or complicated with haematoma.

Causes

Causes of bruising include the following:

- thrombocytopaenia of any cause, such as in leukaemia and marrow aplasia;
- drugs (for example anticoagulants such as warfarin and heparin, steroids and thiazides);
- senile purpura;
- haemophilia;
- blunt injury, such as accidental fall or abuse in children and the elderly.

History and clinical examination

Age should be established, as there is increased risk of bruising in the elderly population. The history should also include detailed enquiry about risk of falls. Specific conditions like COPD, rheumatoid arthritis and asthma should be enquired, as patients with these conditions are also likely to be treated with steroids.

Specific investigations

Full blood cell count
Clotting screen
Antinuclear factor – to rule out vasculitis

ANAEMIA

Anaemia can be defined as a haemoglobin concentration in peripheral blood below the normal range for the sex and age of the patient (Mehta & Hoffbrand 2009), typically less than 13 g/dL in men and less than 11.5 g/dL in women. Commonly, anaemia occurs as a result of blood loss, haemolysis and impaired formation of haemoglobin due to the deficiency of iron, vitamin B_{12} or folate (Mehta & Hoffbrand 2009).

Causes

Causes of anaemia include the following (Mehta & Hoffbrand 2009, Raftery *et al.* 2010):

- drugs, for example non-steroidal anti-inflammatory drugs (NSAIDs), aspirin, warfarin, phenytoin and chloramphenicol;
- bleeding, for example peptic ulcer, colonic polyps and menstrual loss;
- chronic disease, for example rheumatoid arthritis and malignancy;
- iron deficiency, for example in vegans, colonic tumour and elderly patients;
- vitamin B_{12} deficiency, for example because of pernicious anaemia, gastrectomy and malabsorption and in vegans;
- haemolysis, for example mechanical prosthetic valves and autoimmune haemolytic anaemia;
- bone marrow suppression of any cause.

History and clinical examination

History taking and clinical examination should try to establish symptoms suggestive of anaemia and to determine the likely cause. Often, clinical examination is normal. Check for the following:

- pallor – check the skin and conjunctiva;
- tachycardia, murmurs and cardiomegaly – these may be present especially in severe anaemia (haemoglobin < 8 g/dL);
- bruises;
- retinal haemorrhage;
- jaundice – if the primary cause of anaemia is haemolysis;
- chest pain (angina).

Specific investigations

Full blood cell count: the haemoglobin level will confirm the presence or absence of anaemia.

Mean cell volume: low in microcytic anaemia (usually iron deficiency anaemia), normal in anaemia of chronic disease and high in macrocytic anaemia (usually because of alcoholism, vitamin B_{12} and folate deficiency, myxoedema, liver disease and pregnancy).

Serum iron, ferritin, vitamin B_{12} and folate levels: abnormalities can help to identify the cause of anaemia.

If the cause is not uncovered by the history and above-mentioned tests, subsequent investigations may include faecal occult blood, gastroscopy, colonoscopy, barium enema and bone marrow biopsy.

HYPOTENSION

Definition

Hypotension refers to abnormally low BP for the individual. In most people a healthy BP ranges from 90/60 to 120/80 mmHg.

Causes

Its causes are as follows (Jevon 2008):

- heart failure;

- sepsis – causes vasodilation and reduced peripheral resistant and drop in BP;
- hypovolaemia – bleeding (external or internal), dehydration, burns, diuretics, diarrhoea and vomiting;
- anaphylaxis;
- shock, especially in late stage;
- drugs such as anti-hypertensives, opiates, nitrates, diuretics, anaesthetic agents and spinal anaesthesia.

History and clinical examination

Ask about postural dizziness and syncopes. Enquire about a history of IHD, peptic ulcer disease and use of diuretics, beta-blockers, angiotensin-converting enzyme inhibitors and other anti-hypertensives, as well as aspirin and NSAIDs. Enquire about fluid intake and the possibility of dehydration, especially in elderly patients. Trauma, recent surgery or immediate post-operative period may indicate haemorrhage as a cause of hypotension.

Precipitating factors

These depend on the specific cause of hypotension.

Symptoms and signs

Common symptoms include the following:

- dizziness or light-headedness;
- fainting or syncopes – transient loss of consciousness due to reduced cerebral perfusion;
- lethargy;
- headaches and
- seizures.

Clinical signs may include the following (Jevon 2008):

- tachycardia and weak pulse;
- cold peripheries;

- dry oral mucosa and reduced skin turgor;
- signs of heart failure – elevated jugular venous pressure, dyspnoea, leg oedema and bradycardia;
- fever if sepsis is present;
- evidence of haemorrhage and
- normal findings.

Investigations
- A full blood cell count may show anaemia or elevated white blood cells if sepsis is present.
- A clotting screen may show coagulopathy which may be responsible for some hypovolaemic shock due to haemorrhage.
- An ECG may show evidence of MI, heart block or arrhythmia.
- Chest X-ray.
- Blood culture if sepsis is suspected.
- Lying and standing BP can be useful if postural hypotension is suspected. A drop in the systolic BP of 20 mmHg or more when standing is consistent with a diagnosis of postural hypotension.

REFERENCES
Beevers, G., Lip, G. & O'Brien, E. (2007) *ABC of Hypertension*, 5th edn. Blackwell, Oxford.
British Hypertensive Society (2010) http://www.bhsoc.org (accessed 26 May 2010).
Donnelly, R. & London, N. (eds) (2009) *ABC of Arterial & Venous Disease*, 2nd edn. Wiley Blackwell, Oxford.
Gohel, M. & Poskitt, K. (2009) Venous ulceration. In: Donnelly, R. & London, N. (eds) *ABC of Arterial & Venous Disease*, 2nd edn. Wiley Blackwell, Oxford.
Jevon, P. (2008) *Treating the Critically Ill Patient*. Blackwell, Oxford.
Jevon, P. (2009) *ECGs for Nurses*, 2nd edn. Wiley Blackwell, Oxford.
Jevon, P., Humphreys, M. & Ewens, B. (2008) *Nursing Medical Emergency Patients*. Blackwell, Oxford.
Llewelyn, H., Ang, H., Lewis, K. *et al.* (2009) *Oxford Handbook of Clinical Diagnosis*, 2nd edn. Oxford University Press, Oxford.

Mehta, A. & Hoffbrand, V. (2009) *Haematology at a Glance*, 3rd edn. Wiley Blackwell, Oxford.

Raftery, A., Lim, E. & Ostor, A. (2010) *Differential Diagnosis*, 3rd edn. Elsevier, London.

Resuscitation Council UK (2006) *Advanced life Support*, 5th edn. Resuscitation Council UK, London.

Clinical Diagnosis of Symptoms Associated with the Gastrointestinal System

4

Yi-Yang Ng

The aim of this chapter is to understand the clinical diagnosis of symptoms associated with the gastrointestinal (GI) system.

LEARNING OUTCOMES

At the end of this chapter, the reader will be able to discuss the clinical diagnosis of the following symptoms associated with the GI system:

- ❏ nausea and vomiting,
- ❏ abdominal pain,
- ❏ abdominal swelling,
- ❏ haematemesis,
- ❏ ascites,
- ❏ constipation,
- ❏ diarrhoea,
- ❏ intestinal obstruction,
- ❏ melaena,
- ❏ rectal bleeding,
- ❏ jaundice,
- ❏ weight loss,

Clinical Diagnosis, 1st edition. Edited by Phil Jevon.
© 2011 Blackwell Publishing Ltd.

❏ weight gain,
❏ hiccup and
❏ steatorrhoea.

NAUSEA AND VOMITING

Nausea can be defined as a feeling of sickness with an inclination to vomit (it derives from the Greek word *naus* meaning 'ship' and the Latin word *nauseosus* meaning 'seasickness'; Soanes & Stevenson 2006). Vomiting can be defined as ejecting matter from the stomach through the mouth (Soanes & Stevenson 2006).

Causes

There are many causes of nausea and vomiting (Box 4.1; Kinirons & Ellis 2005).

Box 4.1   Causes of nausea and vomiting

GI causes
- Oesophageal obstruction due to cancer – stricture.
- Gastric outlet obstruction due to cancer – pyloric stenosis.
- Large-bowel obstruction due to Crohn's disease bowel cancer – diverticular stricture, sigmoid volvulus.
- Small-bowel obstruction due to Crohn's disease – adhesions, gallstone.
- Acute appendicitis.
- Acute pancreatitis.
- Cholecystitis (inflammation of the gall bladder).
- Gastroenteritis.
- Food poisoning caused by bacteria (such as *Staphylococcus aureus, Bacillus cereus*) and viruses (such as the Norwalk virus).
- Paralytic ileus.
- Volvulus of stomach, caecum or sigmoid.

Intra-abdominal non-GI causes
- Acute inferior myocardial infarction (presented with epigastric pain).
- Renal calculi.
- Pregnancy (including ectopic pregnancy), miscarriage.
- Toxic shock syndrome, pelvic inflammatory disease.

Metabolic causes
- Diabetic ketoacidosis.
- Drugs overdose such as that of digoxin.
- Hypercalcaemia.
- Lead poisoning.

Intracranial causes
- Raised intracranial pressure due to a space-occupying lesion or an intracranial haemorrhage.
- Meningitis.
- Migraine.
- Severe hypertension.
- Acute glaucoma.
- Meniere's disease.
- Labyrinthitis.

History and clinical examination

Causes of vomiting can be identified while taking a thorough history. In cases of intestinal obstruction, the interval between eating and vomiting gives some indication as to the level of obstruction. The contents of the vomitus also help in identifying the level of obstruction. Vomitus consisting of faeces, with abdominal distension and constipation, indicates large-bowel obstruction. Projectile vomiting is classically associated with pyloric obstruction and raised intracranial pressure (Douglas *et al.* 2005). The colour and consistency of the vomit should be noted.

Clinical examination should include the following:

- Measurement of vital signs, as hypotension and tachycardia indicate hypovolaemic shock.
- A raised temperature indicates underlying sepsis.
- The general appearance of a patient tells us how unwell a patient is.
- Cardiovascular system examination of the patient with myocardial infarction may reveal new-onset murmur and signs of acute congestive cardiac failure.
- Thorough abdominal and pelvic examination looking out for signs of localised tenderness and intestinal obstruction.
- Neurological examination, especially when intracranial cause is suspected.

Vomiting is a clinical feature of many clinical conditions. Diagnosis of a particular condition associated with vomiting can be achieved by detailed history taking and thorough clinical examination, guided by appropriate investigations/tests.

Specific investigations

After detailed history taking and clinical examination, the following investigations/tests should be considered to aid diagnosis (Raftery & Lim 2006).

- Full blood cell count, urea and electrolytes: to look for sepsis, the inflammatory process and the state of hydration.
- Inflammatory marker (for example erythrocyte sedimentation rate [ESR] and C-reactive protein [CRP]): to detect the inflammatory process.
- Serum calcium: to detect hypercalcaemia.
- Electrocardiogram: to detect the changes caused by myocardial infarction.
- Blood sugar: to detect hyperglycaemia in diabetic ketoacidosis.
- Urine dipstick: to detect glucose and ketones in diabetic ketoacidosis and haematuria in renal calculus.
- Ultrasound scan of the abdomen: to detect gallstones.
- Chest X-ray: to detect malignancy, pneumonia, bronchiectasis and features of congestive cardiac failure.
- Abdominal X-ray: to detect abnormal dilated bowel loops in intestinal obstruction.
- Pregnancy test: to confirm pregnancy, especially important for women who present with a missed period and abdominal pain.
- Computed tomography (CT) brain scan: useful in suspected causes of raised intracranial pressure.
- Endoscopy (oesophago-gastro-duodenoscopy): to detect peptic ulcer disease and malignancy.
- Audiometry: to detect Meniere's disease and labyrinthitis.

ABDOMINAL PAIN

Pain is an unpleasant feeling of varying degree that is conveyed to the brain by sensory neurons. Tenderness is pain which occurs in response to a stimulus, usually from the clinician, such as pressure by their hand. It is possible for a patient to be lying still without pain and yet have an area of tenderness. The patient feels pain – the health care practitioner elicits tenderness (Browse *et al.* 2005).

Box 4.2   Causes of abdominal pain

Generalised abdominal pain
- Perforation of intra-abdominal organs (such as peptic ulcer or perforation of the small bowel and colon).
- Severe pancreatitis.
- Dissecting aneurysm.

Upper abdominal pain
- Right hypochondriac region – cholecystitis, hepatitis, pyelonephritis, cholangitis, lobar pneumonia.
- Epigastric region – pancreatitis, gastritis, peptic ulcer, inferior myocardial infarction.
- Left hypochondriac region – splenic injury, pyelonephritis, lobar pneumonia.

Central abdominal pain
- Right lumbar region – renal calculus, appendicitis in a high appendix.
- Umbilical region – small-bowel obstruction, ruptured abdominal aortic aneurysm, Crohn's disease.
- Left lumbar region – renal calculus, diverticulitis.

Lower abdominal pain
- Salpingitis, ectopic pregnancy, torsion of or haemorrhage into an ovarian cyst.
- Right iliac fossa – appendicitis, Crohn's disease, Meckel's diverticulitis.
- Supra-pubic region – ruptured uterus, acute urinary retention, cystitis.
- Left iliac fossa – diverticulitis, colitis.

General medical diseases
- Diabetic ketoacidosis.
- Hypercalcaemia.
- Porphyria.
- Malaria.
- Gastroenteritis.

Causes

Most abdominal pain is localised, and a number of causes can cause generalised abdominal pain (Box 4.2; Kinirons & Ellis 2005). A knowledge of intra-abdominal structures with their corresponding regions of the abdomen will help in localising the cause of abdominal pain (Talley & O'Connor 2006).

History and clinical examination

The features of pain must be elicited in any condition in order to aid diagnosis. The features of an abdominal pain that must be elicited include the site, time and mode of onset, severity, nature, progression of pain, duration, relieving factors, aggravating factors, radiation and cause (patient's opinion).

Broadly speaking, abdominal pain can be caused by conditions associated with inflammation and those associated with obstruction of the lumen surrounded by the smooth muscle. Inflammation causes constant pain and persists until the condition subsides. Obstruction to a muscular lumen produces a colic. A colic is a pain which fluctuates in severity at frequent intervals and is griping in nature (for example renal colic). History of recent travelling abroad and intravenous drug injection should be sought in patients with suspected hepatitis presenting with jaundice.

Clinical examination should include the following:

- Measurement of vital signs, as hypotension and tachycardia indicate hypovolaemic shock.
- A raised temperature indicates underlying sepsis.
- The general appearance of a patient tells us how unwell a patient is; the conjunctivae are inspected for pallor in patients with suspected haemorrhage, and jaundice may be observed in patients with hepatitis and pancreatitis due to gallstone impaction.
- Cardiovascular system examination of the patient with myocardial infarction may reveal new-onset murmur and signs of acute congestive cardiac failure.
- Thorough abdominal and pelvic examination to look for sign of localised and generalised tenderness and peritonitis (tenderness, rebound, guarding and absent bowel sound).

A diagnosis of some abdominal pain (for example ruptured abdominal aortic aneurysm, acute cholecystitis, acute appendicitis in a young boy) is achieved by detailed history taking and careful clinical assessment. However, in some conditions that present with abdominal pain, despite focused history taking and clinical assessment, diagnosis can be made only with the help of appropriate investigations/tests.

Specific investigations

After detailed history taking and sound clinical examination, the following investigations/tests may help in establishing the diagnosis:

- Full blood cell count, urea and electrolytes: to look for sepsis, the inflammatory process and the state of hydration.
- Inflammatory marker (for example ESR, CRP): to detect the inflammatory process.
- Electrocardiogram: to detect the changes caused by myocardial infarction.
- Blood sugar: to detect hyperglycaemia in diabetic ketoacidosis.
- Urine dipstick: to detect glucose and ketones in diabetic ketoacidosis and haematuria in renal calculus.
- Urine and stool culture: for suspected infective causes.
- Endoscopy (oesophago-gastro-duodenoscopy): for a patient with suspected peptic ulcer, hiatus hernia.
- Abdominal ultrasound scan: for a patient with suspected gallstone, renal calculus, ovarian cyst.
- Abdominal X-ray: to detect abnormal dilated bowel loops in intestinal obstruction.
- Pregnancy test: to confirm pregnancy, especially important for women who present with a missed period and abdominal pain.
- CT scan of the abdomen: to detect and assess the extent of intra-abdominal pathology.

ABDOMINAL SWELLING

Swelling can be defined as an abnormal enlargement of a part of the body, typically resulting from an accumulation of fluid (Soanes & Stevenson 2006). Abdominal swelling can be localised and generalised.

Causes

The swelling of the abdomen can involve the entire abdomen or affect only certain abdominal regions. It is important to have basic knowledge of intra-abdominal structures with their corresponding regions of the abdomen when assessing localised

---

Box 4.3   Causes of generalised abdominal swelling

- Fat
- Fluid (ascites)
- Flatus (gas)
- Faecal impaction
- Foetus

---

abdominal swellings (Douglas *et al.* 2005). Swellings can also arise from the abdominal wall structures such as the skin, sub-cutaneous fascia or muscles (Kinirons & Ellis 2005). Causes of abdominal swelling are listed in Boxes 4.3 and 4.4.

Box 4.4   Causes of intra-abdominal swelling at different regions

Right iliac fossa swelling
- Caecum: carcinoma, Crohn's disease, tuberculosis
- Appendix: abscess
- Ovary: cyst, carcinoma
- External iliac artery: aneurysm
- Pelvic kidney
- Psoas muscle: abscess

Left iliac fossa swelling
- Sigmoid colon: diverticular disease, carcinoma
- Ovary: cyst, carcinoma
- External iliac artery: aneurysm
- Pelvic kidney
- Psoas muscle: abscess

Hypogastric/supra-pubic swelling
- Sigmoid colon: carcinoma
- Ovary: cyst, carcinoma
- Uterus: fibroid, pregnancy
- Urinary bladder: urinary retention, carcinoma

Epigastric swelling
- Stomach: carcinoma, pyloric stenosis
- Liver: enlarged left lobe (for example carcinoma)
- Gall bladder: mucocele or empyema
- Pancreas: carcinoma, cysts, pseudocyst
- Aorta: aneurysm

Right hypochondriac swelling
- Liver: infection, inflammation, carcinoma, haematological disorder
- Gall bladder: mucocele or empyema
- Colon: carcinoma
- Kidney: hydronephrosis, carcinoma

Left hypochondriac swelling
- Spleen: infection, inflammation, haematological disorder, metabolic disease
- Colon: carcinoma
- Kidney: hydronephrosis, carcinoma

Umbilical region swelling
- Small bowel: carcinoma
- Aorta: aneurysm

Left/right lumbar swelling
- Colon: carcinoma
- Kidney: hydronephrosis, carcinoma

History and clinical examination

A thorough history focusing on the GI and genitourinary symptoms should be enquired. In addition, a history of lethargy, dietary changes and weight loss should be sought when carcinoma is suspected.

Clinical examination should include the following:

- Measurement of vital signs, as hypotension and tachycardia indicate hypovolaemic shock.
- A raised temperature indicates underlying sepsis.
- The general appearance of a patient tells us how unwell a patient is; the conjunctivae are inspected for pallor in patients with suspected haemorrhage, and jaundice may be observed in patients with hepatitis and pancreatitis due to gallstone impaction. Cachexia may indicate underlying malignancy.
- Thorough abdominal and pelvic examination to detect the nature of swelling and signs of tenderness.

A diagnosis of abdominal swelling of any cause can be achieved by detailed and careful history taking with thorough clinical assessment of the abdomen, supplemented by appropriate investigations/tests.

Specific investigations

- Full blood cell count, urea and electrolytes: to look for sepsis, the inflammatory process and the state of hydration.
- Inflammatory marker (for example ESR, CRP): to detect the inflammatory process.
- Endoscopy: for a patient with suspected mass at the upper and/or lower GI tract.
- Abdominal ultrasound scan: for a patient with suspected gallstone, renal calculus, ovarian cyst or localised mass.
- Abdominal X-ray: to assess gas pattern within the abdomen.
- Pregnancy test: to confirm pregnancy, especially important for women who present with a missed period and abdominal pain.
- CT scan of the abdomen: to detect and assess the extent of intra-abdominal mass.

HAEMATEMESIS

Haematemesis can be defined as 'the vomiting of blood'; *haemato* means 'of blood' and *emesis* derives from the Greek word meaning 'vomiting' (Soanes & Stevenson 2006). It is an important feature of upper GI haemorrhage.

Causes

There are various causes of haematemesis, as outlined in Box 4.5 (Kinirons & Ellis 2005).

History and clinical examination

It is important to find out the quantity and nature of the blood vomited, as this will help in identifying the underlying cause. In addition, acute erosions commonly occur in patients taking aspirin or other NSAIDs or following acute alcohol ingestion. Patients may have concurrent melaena.

Clinical examination should include the following:

- Measurement of vital signs, as hypotension and tachycardia indicate hypovolaemic shock.
- The general appearance of a patient tells us how unwell a patient is; the conjunctivae are inspected for pallor in patients

---

Box 4.5   Causes of haematemesis

Swallowed blood from epistaxis, haemoptysis

Bleeding from mouth or throat

Diseases of the oesophagus
- Oesophagitis
- Varices
- Mallory–Weiss tear
- Ulcer
- Foreign body or cancer perforating the oesophagus and aorta

Diseases of the stomach
- Ulcer
- Gastritis
- Carcinoma

Diseases of the duodenum
- Ulcer
- Carcinoma

Clotting disorder
- Thrombocytopenia
- Leukaemia
- Aplastic anaemia
- Haemophilia
- Scurvy
- Chronic liver disease

Drugs
- Anticoagulant and antiplatelet therapy
Non-steroidal anti-inflammatory drugs (NSAIDs), aspirin, phenylbutazone

---

with suspected haemorrhage. Cachexia may indicate underlying malignancy.
- Look out for clinical features of chronic liver disease such as palmar erythema, jaundice, spider naevi and ascites.
- Perform a thorough abdominal examination including digital rectal examination where melaena may be encountered.

Endoscopy of the oesophagus, stomach and duodenum is vital to confirm the exact diagnosis in all cases of significant haematemesis.

Specific investigations
- Full blood count, urea and electrolytes: to look for anaemia, the inflammatory process, the state of hydration and electrolyte balance.

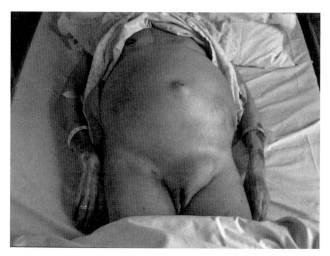

Figure 4.1 Tense ascites with umbilical and left inguinal hernias.

- Inflammatory marker (for example ESR, CRP): to detect the inflammatory process.
- Blood test: to screen for haemophilia and other clotting disorders.
- Endoscopy (oesophago-gastro-duodenoscopy): to identify the source of bleeding and control bleeding.
- Barium study: to identify narrowing of the lumen of the upper GI tract.
- CT scan of the thorax and abdomen: to detect and assess suspected carcinoma at the upper GI tract.

ASCITES

Ascites (Figure 4.1) can be defined as accumulation of fluid in the peritoneal cavity (Soanes & Stevenson 2006).

Causes

Cirrhosis of the liver is the most common cause for ascites (75%), the remainder being a consequence of malignancy (10%), cardiac failure (3%), tuberculosis (2%), pancreatitis (1%) and other rare causes (Moore & Aithal 2006).

Box 4.6 Causes of ascites by the serum ascites to albumin gradient (Moore & Aithal 2006)

High gradient (>1.1 g/dL)
- Cirrhosis
- Nephrotic syndrome
- Cardiac failure

Low gradient (<1.1 g/dL)
- Pancreatitis
- Tuberculosis
- Peritoneal carcinomatosis

The causes of ascites can be classified on the basis of the serum ascites to albumin gradient (Box 4.6; Moore & Aithal 2006).

The pathophysiology of ascites is still poorly understood. Portal hypertension which favours transudation of fluid into peritoneal cavity together with sodium and water retention seen in patients with cirrhosis is implicated in the pathogenesis of non-malignant ascites. In the presence of malignancy, ascites may result from blockage of lymphatic drainage by tumour cells that prevent absorption of intra-peritoneal fluid and protein. In the presence of high protein concentration in many patients with malignant ascites, alteration in vascular permeability results in the development of ascites. Activation renin–angiotensin–aldosterone system is also implicated.

History and clinical examination

The most common cause of ascites is cirrhosis secondary to alcoholism and hepatitis B and C infections. The amount and duration of alcohol consumption and the relevant history of hepatitis B and C exposure (for example the history of travelling abroad, intravenous drug abuse and exchange of body fluid with infected individuals) should be sought.

Clinical examination should include the following:

- The general appearance of a patient tells us how unwell a patient is; cachexia may indicate underlying malignancy and poor nutrition.

- Look out for stigmata of chronic liver disease such as palmar erythema, jaundice and spider naevi.
- Examine the cardiovascular system for features of cardiac failure such as raised jugular venous pressure, enlarged pulsatile liver and pitting ankle oedema.
- Perform a thorough abdominal examination, and detect the extent of ascites by percussion.

The presence of ascites can be confirmed by performing percussion of the abdomen during clinical assessment. Abdominal paracentesis is commonly used to ascertain the underlying cause of ascites and to provide symptomatic relief of massive ascites.

Specific investigations

- Full blood cell count, urea and electrolytes and liver function tests: to look for the infective or inflammatory process, the state of hydration and electrolyte balance and the extent of liver function derangement.
- Inflammatory marker (for example ESR, CRP): to detect the inflammatory process.
- Blood test for clotting screen: this will be abnormal in patients with cirrhosis.
- Blood test for viral hepatitis serology: to find out if this is the underlying cause for cirrhosis.
- Urine dipstick: a large amount of protein may suggest nephrotic syndrome.
- CT scan of the abdomen: to assess intra-abdominal malignancy and the extent of cirrhosis.
- Abdominal paracentesis: to drain ascitic fluid for symptomatic relief of ascites and to perform ascitic fluid analysis.

CONSTIPATION

Constipation can literally be defined as difficulty emptying the bowels, usually associated with hardened faeces (derived from the Latin words *con* meaning 'together' and *stipare* meaning 'press' or 'cram'; Soanes & Stevenson 2006). For medical purposes, constipation is defined as having a bowel movement fewer than three times per week (Douglas *et al*. 2005). The stools are usually hard, dry, small in size and difficult to eliminate. Sometimes, people who are constipated find it painful to have a bowel movement and often experience straining, bloating and the sensation of a full bowel. Normal stool elimination may be three times a day or three times a week.

Causes

Constipation is a symptom, not a disease. Almost everyone experiences constipation at some point in their lives, and a poor diet typically is the cause. There are other causes of constipation, listed in Box 4.7.

Box 4.7   Causes of constipation

Acute intestinal obstruction
- In the lumen
  - Gallstone ileus
  - Faecal impaction
  - Food bolus
- In the wall
  - Crohn's disease
  - Tuberculous stricture
  - Diverticular disease of the colon
  - Tumour of the colon
- Outside the wall
  - Adhesions and bands
  - Strangulated hernia
  - Intussusception
  - Volvulus

Painful anal conditions
- Fissure in ano
- Thrombosed piles

Adynamic bowel
- Hirschsprung's disease
- Spinal cord injury or disease
- Myxoedema

Drugs
- codeine phosphate, morphine, iron supplements and anti- Parkinson's drugs

Irritable bowel syndrome

History and clinical examination

Dietary and drug history is important. Some people think they are constipated if they do not have a bowel movement every day. Therefore, it is important to clarify what constipation means to patients, as bowel habit varies among individuals. It is crucial to elicit other symptoms (for example vomiting, change in bowel habit, weight loss) associated with constipation, which may well suggest an underlying organic cause.

Clinical examination should include the following:

- The general appearance of a patient tells us how unwell a patient is; pallor and cachexia may indicate underlying malignancy and poor nutrition.
- Look for clinical features of hypothyroidism, such as dry skin, puffy face and hands, coarse hair, hoarse and husky voice and slow tendon reflexes.
- Perform a thorough abdominal examination and digital rectal examination to detect perineal, anal canal and rectal pathology.

Not all patients with constipation have poor diet, and it is important not to overlook organic cause(s) of constipation which can be achieved by detailed history taking, thorough clinical examination and appropriate investigation.

Specific investigations

- Full blood cell count: to detect anaemia in patients with colorectal cancer presented with chronic blood loss.
- Inflammatory marker (for example ESR, CRP): to detect the inflammatory process.
- Thyroid function test: to detect hypothyroidism.
- Barium enema X-ray: to view the rectum, colon and lower part of the small bowel to locate problems.
- Abdominal X-ray: to detect faecal loading and abnormal gas pattern in the bowel.
- CT scan of the abdomen: to detect colorectal malignancy and the extent of the disease.
- Endoscopy (colonoscopy or flexible sigmoidoscopy): to directly view the rectum, colon and lower part of the small bowel and allow biopsy of the suspicious area.

DIARRHOEA

Diarrhoea can be defined as a condition in which faeces are discharged from the bowels frequently and in liquid form (from the Greek word *diarrhoia* meaning 'flow through'; Soanes & Stevenson 2006).

Normal stool elimination may be three times a day or three times a week. It should be borne in mind that the patient's and the clinician's perception of bowel function may be quite different. Thus, it is important to make sure that both the patient and the clinician are talking about the same thing.

Causes

The causes of diarrhoea can be classified on the basis of the general features, frequency, consistency and amount of stools passed (Box 4.8; Llewelyn *et al.* 2006).

Box 4.8 Causes of diarrhoea

Recurrent diarrhoea without blood in stools
- Irritable bowel syndrome
- Malabsorption due to coeliac disease, lactose intolerance and pancreatic disease
- Drug induced (laxative, magnesium alkalis, antibiotics)
- Faecal impaction with overflow
- Thyrotoxicosis
- Diabetic autonomic neuropathy

Recurrent diarrhoea with blood (and mucus)
- Crohn's disease
- Ulcerative colitis
- Colorectal carcinoma
- Diverticular disease

Watery diarrhoea
- Traveller's diarrhoea
- Enterotoxigenic *Escherichia coli*
- *Vibrio cholerae*
- Rota and Norwalk viruses

Acute bloody diarrhoea
- Shigella dysentery
- *Campylobacter* enteritis
- Enteroinvasive *E. Coli*
- Enterohaemorrhagic *E. Coli* 0157
- *Entamoeba histolytica*

History and clinical examination

Ask the history of recent travelling for patients presenting with infective diarrhoea. Unexplained weight loss, pallor and change in bowel habit may indicate underlying colorectal malignancy. Ask about symptoms of hyperthyroidism, such as irritability, palpitation, heat intolerance and tremor.

Clinical examination should include the following:

- Measurement of vital signs, as a raised temperature may indicate underlying sepsis. Hypotension and tachycardia indicate hypovolaemic shock.
- The general appearance of a patient tells us how unwell a patient is; the conjunctivae are inspected for pallor in patients with suspected blood loss. Cachexia may indicate underlying malignancy. Sweaty palms, irregular heart rate and agitation may suggest hyperthyroidism.
- Perform a thorough abdominal examination including digital rectal examination where the consistency and nature of the stool can be examined.

Endoscopic examination should be considered in patients presenting with bloody diarrhoea when infective causes have been ruled out.

Specific investigations

- Full blood cell count, urea and electrolytes: to look for anaemia, the inflammatory process, the state of hydration and electrolyte balance.
- Inflammatory marker (for example ESR, CRP): to detect the inflammatory process.
- Blood sugar: elevated level (above the normal range) indicates diabetes mellitus.
- Coeliac screen: to detect coeliac disease.
- Thyroid function test: to detect hyperthyroidism.
- Stool microscopy and culture: to detect infective cause(s) of diarrhoea.
- Barium enema X-ray: to view the rectum, colon and lower part of the small bowel to locate problems.

- Endoscopy (colonoscopy or flexible sigmoidoscopy): to directly view the rectum, colon and lower part of the small bowel and allow biopsy of the suspicious area.
- CT scan of the abdomen: to detect and assess suspected colorectal carcinoma.

DYSPHAGIA

Dysphagia can be defined as difficulty in swallowing (from the Greek words *dys* meaning 'difficult' and *phagos* meaning 'eat'; Soanes & Stevenson 2006). Odynophagia describes pain on swallowing.

Causes

Dysphagia can be caused by a disease process involving the lumen and the inside and outside of the wall of the throat, oesophagus and stomach (Box 4.9; Talley & O'Connor 2006).

History and clinical examination

It is important to assess the severity of dysphagia on the basis of the ability to swallow solids and liquids. If the patient

---

Box 4.9   Causes of dysphagia

In the lumen
- Reflux oesophagitis with stricture formation
- Carcinoma of the oesophagus or the stomach
- Pharyngeal or oesophageal web
- Pharyngeal pouch
- Foreign body

In the wall
- Diffuse oesophageal spasm
- Achalasia
- Bulbar/pseudobulbar palsy
- Myasthenia gravis
- Scleroderma

Outside the wall
- Enlargement of the thyroid
- Carcinoma of the thymus
- Enlargement of mediastinal lymph nodes

---

complains of difficulty initiating swallowing with fluid regurgitating into the nose or choking, this suggests that the cause of dysphagia is at the pharynx (throat). If the patient complains that solids and liquids stick, then a motor disorder such as achalasia or diffuse oesophageal spasm is most likely.

Clinical examination should include the following:

- The general appearance of a patient tells us how unwell a patient is; the conjunctivae are inspected for pallor in patients with suspected blood loss. Cachexia may indicate underlying malignancy.
- Perform a thorough neurological and cranial nerve examination in patients with suspected neurological disorder such as myasthenia gravis and bulbar and pseudobulbar palsy.
- Perform a thorough abdominal examination.

Cancer is the most important differential diagnosis in the context of dysphagia; the main tool for this investigation is endoscopy.

Specific investigations
- Full blood cell count: to detect anaemia due to chronic blood loss.
- Tensilon test and anti-acetylcholine antibody: to diagnose myasthenia gravis.
- Barium swallow: to detect luminal pathology and demonstrate abnormal peristalsis.
- Oesophageal manometry: to demonstrate the abnormal pressure profile of the oesophagus.
- Endoscopy (oesophageal-gastro-duodenoscopy): to visualise abnormality along the throat, oesophagus and stomach and to allow biopsy of the suspicious area.
- CT scan of the thorax: to detect mediastinal malignancy and enlarged lymph nodes.

INTESTINAL OBSTRUCTION
Intestinal obstruction is a blockage of the small intestine or the colon that prevents food and fluid from passing through.

Box 4.10 Causes of intestinal obstruction

In the lumen
- Gallstone ileus
- Faecal impaction
- Food bolus

In the wall
- Crohn's disease
- Tuberculous stricture
- Diverticular disease of the colon
- Tumour of the colon

Outside the wall
- Adhesions and bands
- Strangulated hernia
- Intussusception
- Volvulus

Causes

Intestinal obstruction can be caused by a disease process affecting the lumen, the wall and the outside of the wall of the intestine (Box 4.10; Kinirons & Ellis 2005).

History and clinical examination

A history of previous abdominal surgery (adhesions) and change in bowel habit (possible colorectal cancer) should be sought. The cardinal features of intestinal obstruction are colicky abdominal pain, vomiting, abdominal distension and absolute constipation.

Clinical examination should include the following:

- The general appearance of a patient tells us how unwell a patient is; pallor and cachexia may indicate underlying malignancy.
- Examine the groins for hernia.
- Perform a thorough abdominal examination to detect signs of abdominal obstruction and digital rectal examination to detect perineal, anal canal and rectal pathology.

A history and sound clinical assessment are sufficient in most circumstances in diagnosing intestinal obstruction prior to further investigations/tests to detect underlying cause. Prompt diagnosis of intestinal obstruction is crucial, as delayed diagnosis may lead to perforation of the bowel, resulting in generalised peritonitis.

Specific investigations
- Full blood cell count: to detect anaemia and the inflammatory and infective process.
- Urea and electrolytes: to detect fluid and electrolyte disturbance due to vomiting because of intestinal obstruction.
- Inflammatory marker (for example ESR, CRP): to detect the inflammatory process.
- Abdominal X-ray: to detect abnormal dilated bowel loop and gas pattern.
- Water-soluble contrast X-ray: to detect the mechanical cause and level of intestinal obstruction.
- Endoscopy (colonoscopy or flexible sigmoidoscopy): to directly view the rectum, colon and lower part of the small bowel and allow biopsy of the suspicious area once the obstruction has resolved.
- CT scan of the abdomen: to detect the nature and level of intestinal obstruction.

MELAENA
Melaena can be defined as the production of dark sticky faeces containing blood (from the Greek word *melas* meaning 'black'; Soanes & Stevenson 2006). It is passing of black bowel motion due to haemorrhage which has occurred in the upper GI tract. Melaena stools are black and tarry, with a sticky consistency, making it difficult to flush them down the toilet (Kinirons & Ellis 2005).

Causes
Melaena is most commonly due to bleeding from the stomach or duodenum and rarely from the oesophagus (Box 4.11; Llewelyn *et al.* 2006).

Box 4.11   Causes of melaena

Oesophagus
- Carcinoma
- Ingestion of a corrosive
- Varices
- Hiatus hernia
- Mallory–Weiss tear

Stomach
- Carcinoma
- Erosion
- Ulcer
- Hiatus hernia

Duodenum
- ulcer

Small bowel
- Meckel's diverticulum
- Angiodysplasia
- Crohn's disease

History and clinical examination

Acute erosions commonly occur in patients taking aspirin or other NSAIDs. Patients may have concurrent haematemesis. Apart from melaena, black or dark stools may occur after taking iron preparations, bismuth preparations or liquorice or following ingestion of black cherries, bilberries or red wine in large amounts (Raftery & Lim 2006).

Clinical examination should include the following:

- Measurement of vital signs, as hypotension and tachycardia indicate hypovolaemic shock.
- The general appearance of a patient tells us how unwell a patient is; the conjunctivae are inspected for pallor in patients with suspected haemorrhage. Cachexia may indicate underlying malignancy.
- Perform a thorough abdominal examination to detect areas of tenderness and mass; also perform digital rectal examination where melaena may be confirmed.

Specific investigations
- Full blood cell count, urea and electrolytes: to look for anaemia, the inflammatory process, the state of hydration and electrolyte balance.
- Inflammatory marker (for example ESR, CRP): to detect the inflammatory process.
- Faecal occult blood: especially in patients with iron deficiency anaemia with suspected upper GI haemorrhage.
- Endoscopy (oesophago-gastro-duodenoscopy): to identify the source of bleeding and control bleeding.

Endoscopy of the oesophagus, stomach and duodenum is vital in all cases of melaena.

RECTAL BLEEDING
Rectal bleeding, also known as haematochezia, refers to the passage of bright red blood via the rectum (Douglas *et al.* 2005).

Causes
Rectal bleeding can be due to bleeding from anywhere along the lower GI tract, namely the colon, rectum and anus (Box 4.12; Kinirons & Ellis 2005).

Box 4.12   Causes of rectal bleeding

General causes
- Clotting disorder
- Anticoagulants

Colonic causes
- Diverticular disease
- Infective
- Inflammatory bowel disease (Crohn's disease and ulcerative colitis)
- Angiodysplasia
- Ischaemia
- Neoplasm (adenoma and carcinoma)
- Polyps

Rectal causes
- Infective
- Inflammatory bowel disease

- Solitary rectal ulcer
- Trauma
- Neoplasm (adenoma, carcinoma and malignant melanoma)

Anal causes
- Haemorrhoids
- Fissure in ano
- Anal fistula
- Trauma
- Malignancy (squamous carcinoma, malignant melanoma, adenocarcinoma and Paget's disease)

History and clinical examination

Ask about unexplained weight loss, change in bowel habit and lethargy in suspected cases of malignancy. The presence of bright red blood not mixed with stools suggests bleeding from haemorrhoids or anal fissure. Blood mixing with stools suggests blood arising above the anorectum (such as diverticular disease, carcinoma of the colon).

Clinical examination should include the following:

- Measurement of vital signs, as hypotension and tachycardia indicate hypovolaemic shock.
- The general appearance of a patient tells us how unwell a patient is; the conjunctivae are inspected for pallor in patients with suspected haemorrhage. Cachexia may indicate underlying malignancy.
- A thorough abdominal examination including digital rectal examination where pathology arising from the lower rectum and anal canal can be felt and, also, to confirm the presence of blood in the rectum.
- Proctoscopy should be carried out in patients with a history suggesting haemorrhoids.

Specific investigations

- Full blood count, urea and electrolytes: to look for anaemia, the inflammatory process, the state of hydration and electrolyte balance.
- Inflammatory marker (for example ESR, CRP): to detect the inflammatory process.

- Clotting screen: to detect clotting disorder.
- Barium enema X-ray: to view the rectum, colon and lower part of the small bowel to locate the pathology.
- Endoscopy (colonoscopy or flexible sigmoidoscopy): to directly view the rectum, colon and lower part of the small bowel and allow biopsy of the suspicious area.

JAUNDICE

Jaundice is the presence of excess bilirubin being deposited in the sclera and/or skin, resulting in yellow discoloration (Raftery & Lim 2006).

Causes

The causes of jaundice can be divided into prehepatic, hepatic and obstructive (cholestatic) jaundice (Box 4.13; Douglas *et al.* 2005).

Box 4.13   Causes of jaundice

Prehepatic jaundice
- Congenital
  - Gilbert's disease
  - Crigler–Najjar syndrome
- Haemolysis
  - Hereditary spherocytosis
  - Sickle cell disease
  - G6PD deficiency
  - Thalassaemia
  - Malaria
  - Autoimmune
  - Hypersplenism

Hepatic jaundice
- Viral hepatitis
  - Hepatitis A, B, C
  - Epstein–Barr virus
  - Cytomegalovirus
- Drugs (for example paracetamol, halothane)
- Toxins (for example carbon tetrachloride)
- Autoimmune
- End-stage liver disease
  - Alcohol
  - Cirrhosis

- ○ Haemochromatosis
- ○ Wilson's disease

Obstructive (cholestatic) jaundice
- Gallstones
- Cholangiocarcinoma
- Stricture
- Cholangitis
- Sclerosing cholangitis
- Carcinoma of the head of the pancreas
- Carcinoma of the ampulla of Vater
- Enlarged lymph nodes in porta hepatis
- Mirizzi syndrome

History and clinical examination

Ask about family history of blood disorder, racial origin, history of anaemia and drug history in prehepatic jaundice. Ask about contact with jaundice, occupation, travel, alcohol, sexual activity, drugs, previous episodes of jaundice and blood transfusion in hepatic jaundice. Ask about a history of abdominal pain (biliary colic), dark urine, pale stools and itching in obstructive jaundice.

Clinical examination should include the following:

- Look at the general appearance to detect the extent of jaundice; pallor may suggest underlying anaemia; cachexia may indicate malignancy; look for pin-track marks along the vein in suspected intravenous drug abuser (viral hepatitis).
- Check vital signs for raised temperature which may indicate underlying sepsis.
- Perform a thorough abdominal examination including looking out for features of chronic liver disease such as palmar erythema, spider naevi, bruising and ascites.

Remember to ask questions specific to prehepatic, hepatic and obstructive jaundice. Sometimes, despite detailed clinical history and clinical examination, the cause of jaundice may not be clear, and this is when specific investigations/tests will be of help.

Specific investigations
- Full blood cell count: to detect anaemia and the inflammatory and infective process.

- Coomb's test: positive in autoimmune haemolysis.
- Blood film: to detect abnormal morphology of red blood cells and malarial plasmodium.
- Liver function test: raised bilirubin in all cases of jaundice; raised transaminases in obstructive jaundice but markedly raised in hepatic jaundice; raised alkaline phosphatase in hepatic jaundice but markedly raised in obstructive jaundice.
- Urinalysis: raised bilirubin in hepatic and obstructive jaundice; raised urobilinogen in both prehepatic and hepatic jaundice.
- Viral antibodies: to detect hepatitis A, B and C, cytomegalovirus and the Epstein–Barr virus.
- Serum copper and ceruloplasmin: reduced in Wilson's disease.
- Serum iron: raised in haemochromatosis.
- Ultrasound scan of the abdomen: to detect gallstones and dilated biliary tree.
- CT scan of the abdomen: to detect carcinoma of the head of the pancreas.
- Endoscopic retrograde cholangiopancreatography: to detect the presence of abnormality at the bile duct and allow biopsy of the suspicious area. Gallstone retrieval at the common bile duct can be performed under the same procedure if appropriate.

WEIGHT LOSS

Weight loss is the loss of body mass, characterised by loss of body fat and skeletal muscle. Unintentional weight loss may be a manifestation of underlying illness.

Causes

The causes of weight loss include systemic illness, endocrinological disease, infective disease and psychiatric illness (Box 4.14; Kinirons & Ellis 2005).

Box 4.14   Causes of weight loss

Systemic illness
- Malignancy
- Chronic cardiorespiratory diseases

- Malabsorption
- Liver failure
- Renal failure

Endocrinological disease
- Hyperthyroidism
- Diabetes mellitus
- Addison's disease

Infective disease
- Tuberculosis
- HIV
- Helminth (worm) infection

Psychiatric illness
- Depression
- Anorexia nervosa

History and clinical examination

Ask about dietary history, and enquiry should be undertaken concerning the perception of body image in patients with suspected eating disorder. Ask about symptoms of chronic cardiorespiratory disease such as shortness of breath, orthopnoea, paroxysmal nocturnal dypsnoea and night sweats. Classical features of thyrotoxicosis are tremor, heat intolerance, palpitations and diarrhoea. Risk factors for HIV should be asked, which include sexual history and intravenous drug use.

Clinical examination should include the following:

- Check the clinical appearance for pallor which may indicate anaemia due to underlying malignancy; check for dry skin and hair changes seen in anorexia nervosa, and measure the body mass index; enlarged lymph nodes may be detected in advanced malignancy, tuberculosis and HIV.
- Look for signs of hyperthyroidism such as tremor, sweaty palms, atrial fibrillation and eye signs (proptosis, chemosis and ophthalmoplegia) of Grave's disease
- Perform thorough clinical examination of the cardiorespiratory system and abdomen.

It is important to establish actual weight loss by detailed history taking. Clinical examination and specific investigations are useful in establishing the underlying cause of weight loss in many circumstances.

Specific investigations

- Full blood cell count: to detect anaemia in chronic disease, malabsorption and malignancy.
- Urea and electrolytes: raised urea and creatinine in renal failure; decreased sodium and increased potassium in Addison's disease.
- Liver function test: raised bilirubin, transaminases and decreased albumin in liver failure.
- Blood glucose: raised (above the normal range) in diabetes mellitus.
- Thyroid function test: to detect hyperthyroidism.
- Chest X-ray: to detect changes due to cardiac failure and abnormality may be seen in tuberculosis and malignancy.
- Echocardiography: to detect cardiac failure.
- Endoscopy (upper and lower GI tract): to detect malignancy/inflammation.
- CT scan of the thorax and abdomen: to detect malignancy.
- Stool microscopy and culture: to detect the presence of helminths and their ova.
- HIV antibodies: to diagnose HIV infection.

WEIGHT GAIN

Weight gain is an increase in body weight. This can be due to an increase in muscle mass, fat or excess fluid accumulation (Kinirons & Ellis 2005).

Causes

Causes of weight gain include pregnancy, organ enlargement, excess fat, excess fluid retention and excess muscle (Box 4.15; Raftery & Lim 2006).

Box 4.15   Causes of weight gain

Pregnancy

Organ enlargement: Polycystic ovarian syndrome

Excess fat
- Cushing's syndrome
- Hypothyroidism
- Hypothalamic disease
- Obesity

Excess fluid retention
- Cardiac failure
- Renal failure – nephrotic syndrome
- Liver failure – ascites
- Lymphatic obstruction

Excess muscle
- Growth hormone
- Androgenic steroids
- Athletes, for example weightlifters

History and clinical examination

Ask about the possibility of pregnancy and any changes in dietary habit. Ask about drug history, especially consumption of anabolic steroid and growth hormone. Ask about excess hair growth, acne, thick skin and muscle weakness for Cushing's syndrome. Lethargy, cold intolerance, dry hair and skin and menorrhagia are typical of hypothyroidism. Hirsutism, menstrual irregularities and insulin resistance can be found in patients with polycystic ovarian syndrome.

Clinical examination should include the following:

- Check the general appearance for distribution of body fat, as truncal obesity with proximal muscle wasting is classic of patients with Cushing's syndrome. Loss of the outer third of the eyebrows is a feature of hypothyroidism.
- Perform a thorough clinical assessment of the abdomen, and look for gravid uterus and ascites.
- Check for signs of cardiac failure, such as raised jugular venous pressure, enlarged pulsatile liver, pitting ankle oedema and bibasal crepitations.

Obesity is becoming common in the Western society (Kinirons & Ellis 2005), and it is due to an energy intake in excess of energy expenditure. Diagnosis can usually be achieved with detailed history taking and clinical assessment. Diagnosis of other causes of weight gain may require specific investigations.

Specific investigations
- Full blood cell count: to detect anaemia of chronic illness.
- Urea and electrolytes: raised urea and creatinine in renal impairment; low potassium level seen in Cushing's syndrome.
- Liver function test: to detect liver failure.
- Thyroid function test: to screen for thyroid disease.
- Pregnancy test: to confirm pregnancy.
- Urine dipstick: proteinuria seen in nephrotic syndrome and possibly haematuria in renal disease.
- Random cortisol level: raised level may suggest Cushing's syndrome.
- 24-h urinary free-cortisol level: raised in Cushing's syndrome.
- Echocardiography: to detect cardiac failure.
- Ultrasound scan of the abdomen and pelvis: to detect renal disorder and polycystic ovaries.
- CT/magnetic resonance imaging (MRI) scan of the head: to detect hypothalamic disease.

HICCUP
Hiccup is caused by sudden involuntary contraction of both the diaphragm and the external intercostal muscles associated with rapid closure of the glottis.

Causes
Gastric distension (causing diaphragmatic irritation) after rapid ingestion of alcohol, air or food is the most common cause of hiccup. This is usually self-limiting. Causes of persistent hiccup include phrenic nerve irritation, diaphragmatic irritation and diseases of the central nervous system (Box 4.16; Raftery & Lim 2006).

Box 4.16   Causes of persistent hiccup

Phrenic nerve irritation
- Lung tumour
- Oesophageal carcinoma
- Thoracic surgery

Diaphragmatic irritation
- Subphrenic abscess

- Diaphragmatic hernia
- Lower lobe pneumonia
- Empyema

Central nervous system diseases
- Meningitis
- Encephalitis
- Tumours
- Intracranial haemorrhage
- Brainstem stroke

Others
- Hysterical
- Renal failure
- Drugs such as benzodiazepines and short-acting barbiturates

History and clinical examination

The causes of hiccups are mainly the result of diseases of the central nervous system, respiratory system and alimentary tract; the history should focus on these areas. Ask about drug history, as certain drugs, as those outlined earlier, may cause persistent hiccups.

Clinical examination should include the following:

- Measure vital signs, as swinging pyrexia may indicate underlying pus collection as seen in empyema and subphrenic abscess.
- Conduct a thorough examination of the respiratory system, looking for changes due to consolidation and pleural effusion.
- Carry out an abdominal examination looking for an area of tenderness.
- Perform neurological examination (Douglas *et al.* 2005) including checking for focal neurological deficit, Kernig's sign (pain on extension of the knee from a flexed hip and knee) and Brudzinski's sign (flexion of the neck produces flexion of the hip and knee).

Persistent hiccup must not be overlooked; the underlying cause should be sought with detailed history, careful clinical examination and appropriate investigation(s).

Specific investigations

- Full blood cell count: to detect anaemia in chronic illness. Raised white cell count is seen in infection.
- Urea and electrolytes: raised urea and creatinine in renal failure.
- Inflammatory marker (for example ESR, CRP): to detect the inflammatory process.
- Chest X-ray: to detect consolidation, abnormalities of the hilar and changes suggestive of carcinoma. Elevation of the diaphragm may be due to phrenic nerve palsy.
- CT scan of the thorax: to detect bronchial carcinoma and empyema.
- CT scan of the abdomen: to detect intra-abdominal abscess.
- CT/MRI scan of the head: to detect intracranial haemorrhage, infarction and tumour of the brain. Cortical swelling may be seen with encephalitis.
- Lumbar puncture: to detect meningitis.

STEATORRHOEA

Steatorrhoea is excess fat in the faeces due to reduced absorption of fat from the intestine (Soanes & Stevenson 2006).

Causes

There are many causes of steatorrhoea, including intestinal mucoal disease, lipase deficiency and bile deficiency (Box 4.17; Raftery & Lim 2006).

Box 4.17 Causes of steatorrhoea

Intestinal mucosal disease
- Resection of the ileum
- Coeliac disease
- Crohn's disease

Lipase deficiency
- Impaired secretion (for example chronic pancreatitis)
- Inactivation (for example excessive gastric acid in Zollinger–Ellison syndrome)

Bile deficiency
- Underproduction (for example liver disease)
- Obstruction of the bile duct (for example obstructive jaundice)
- Increased degradation (for example bacterial overgrowth)

History and clinical examination

The stools are generally bulky, greasy, malodorous and pale in colour in steatorrhoea. Ask about a history of previous abdominal surgery that involved ileal resection; abdominal pain and rectal bleeding in Crohn's disease and epigastric pain with dyspepsia exacerbated by food may be seen in Zollinger–Ellison syndrome. A history of recurrent epigastric pain radiating to the back may suggest chronic pancreatitis.

Clinical examination should include the following:

- Perform a general inspection looking for jaundice due to bile duct obstruction, abnormal rash such as dermatitis herpetiformis in coeliac disease and erythema nodosum seen in Crohn's disease.
- Conduct a thorough abdominal examination and check for hepatomegaly seen in liver disease. Also check perineum for perianal abscesses and fistulae which may be present in Crohn's disease.

Steatorrhoea is a feature of many causes, as mentioned. It is important to ask relevant history, combined with sound clinical examination and appropriate investigations in order to diagnose the underlying cause of the clinical feature.

Specific investigations

- Full blood cell count: to detect anaemia due to chronic illness and elevated white blood cell count seen in the inflammatory and infective process.
- Inflammatory marker (for example ESR, CRP): to detect the inflammatory process.
- Amylase: usually not elevated in chronic pancreatitis but may be raised in recurrent acute attacks.

- Liver function test: Raised bilirubin, alkaline phosphatase and transaminases in obstructive jaundice; decreased albumin in malabsorption syndrome.
- Antigliadin, antiendomysial and antireticulin antibodies: to detect coeliac disease.
- Serum gastrin assay: to detect Zollinger–Ellison syndrome.
- Abdominal X-ray: to detect calcification in chronic pancreatitis.
- CT scan of the abdomen: to detect liver disease.
- Small-bowel enema: to detect strictures, fistulae and skip lesions caused by Crohn's disease.
- Colonoscopy: to detect Crohn's disease of the large bowel.
- Jejunal biopsy: to detect changes due to coeliac disease.

REFERENCES
Beckingham, I. (ed.) (2001) *ABC of Liver, Pancreas and Gall Bladder*. BMJ Books, London.

Browse, N.L., Black, J., Burnand, K.G. *et al.* (2005) *Browse's Introduction to the Symptoms and Signs of Surgical Diseases*, 4th edn. Hodder Education, London.

Douglas, G., Nicol, F. & Robertson, C. (2005) *MacLeod's Clinical Examination*, 11th edn. Elsevier Churchill Livingstone, London.

Kinirons, M. & Ellis, H. (2005) *French's Index of Differential Diagnosis: An A–Z*, 14th edn. Hodder Arnold, London.

Llewelyn, H., Ang, H.A., Lewis, K. *et al.* (2006) *Oxford Handbook of Clinical Diagnosis*, 1st edn. Oxford University Press, Oxford.

Moore, K.P. & Aithal, G.P. (2006) Guidelines on the management of ascites in cirrhosis. *Gut* **55**, 1–12.

Raftery, A.T. & Lim, E. (2006) *Churchill's Pocketbook of Differential Diagnosis*, 2nd edn. Elsevier Churchill Livingstone, London.

Soanes, C. & Stevenson, A. (eds) (2006) *Concise Oxford English Dictionary*, 11th edn. Oxford University Press, Oxford.

Talley, N.J. & O'Connor, S. (2006) *Clinical Examination: A Systematic Guide to Physical Diagnosis*, 5th edn. Elsevier Churchill Livingstone, Marrickville, New South Wales, Australia.

Clinical Diagnosis of Symptoms Associated with the Neurological System

5

Kathryn Blakey and Gareth Walters

The aim of this chapter, is to understand the clinical diagnosis of symptoms associated with the neurological system.

LEARNING OUTCOMES

At the end of this chapter the reader will be able to discuss the clinical diagnosis of the following symptoms associated with the neurological system:

❏ headache,
❏ syncope,
❏ dizziness,
❏ seizure,
❏ tremor,
❏ hemiplegia,
❏ acute confusion and
❏ reduced conscious level and coma.

HEADACHE

Headache describes pain felt in the head region, including behind the eyes and ears, on top of the head and at the back of the neck (occipital pain). An important skill is being able to identify those who may have a serious underlying cause. This is normally possible only by taking a thorough history. Using an

Clinical Diagnosis, 1st edition. Edited by Phil Jevon.
© 2011 Blackwell Publishing Ltd.

approach to history taking such as TINA (timing, influences, nature and associations) can aid diagnosis.

Headache is a very common problem, experienced by almost everybody at some point. It is one of the most common presentations in medicine and usually does not indicate serious intracranial disease. For example, tension headaches are experienced by 90% of the population at some time. Headache can be a non-specific symptom that accompanies systemic disease, such as viral infection and hypoglycaemia (Kumar & Clark 2005)

Causes

The more common causes of headache are shown in Table 5.1. The associated clinical features are usually more important than tests in making an initial diagnosis.

History and clinical examination

Timing

Sudden-onset, severe, occipital headache that is often described as the 'worst headache ever' (thunder-clap headache) is suggestive of a subarachnoid haemorrhage, a bleed into the space below the arachnoid membrane surrounding the brain. Sudden-onset headache following a significant head injury, or even a trivial injury in the elderly patients taking anticoagulants, may indicate extradural or subdural haemorrhage (bleeds above or below the dural membrane). Most headaches post-injury are benign, as part of a concussion syndrome, and are therefore not associated with any significant pathology. Recurrent acute headaches that come on over a few minutes and gradually intensify may also be migraine or cluster headaches. A frontal headache that develops gradually over days to weeks and is worse in the morning, or on straining and coughing, raises the suspicion of raised intracranial pressure (ICP) because of a space-occupying lesion (SOL) such as a tumour or an abscess. Raised ICP also causes vomiting and, eventually, drowsiness due to compression of the brainstem.

Influences

Photophobia (dislike of bright light) is seen with headaches associated with meningitis and migraine. Some patients who

Table 5.1 Common causes of headache, showing associated symptoms and signs.

Differential diagnosis	Associated symptoms and signs
Migraine	Visual aura lasting 10–30 min (flashing lights, loss of vision); occasionally speech disturbance, hemiplegia
	Accompanied by nausea and vomiting
	Normal conscious level, photophobia, usually no focal neurological signs
Meningitis	Preceding respiratory tract or ear infection, fever, vomiting, generally unwell
	Non-blanching petechial rash, photophobia, neck stiffness, reduced conscious level
Subarachnoid haemorrhage	Neck pain and stiffness, nausea and vomiting
	If severe, then seizures, reduced conscious level, focal neurological signs and pupil abnormalities
SOL causing raised ICP; e.g. tumour, abscess, chronic subdural haematoma	Progressive neurological symptoms, e.g. unsteady gait, visual disturbance, progressive limb weakness, personality change); nausea and vomiting, seizures
	Swollen optic disc on fundoscopy (papilloedema), pupil abnormalities, focal neurological signs and reduced conscious level; reduced pulse and raised blood pressure (Cushing response)
Temporal arteritis (giant-cell arteritis)	Jaw pain, scalp tenderness, altered vision, upper limb loss of function
	Tender palpable temporal arteries, proximal upper limb weakness, optic nerve atrophy
Cluster headache	Unilateral eye pain – pain lasts 20–60 min, in clusters typically daily for a few weeks or months
	Unilateral facial flushing, red and watery eyes, nasal secretions; no abnormal neurological signs
Tension headache	Associated with emotional stress and anxiety, continuous loud noise or fumes
	No abnormal neurological signs

suffer with migraine are also aware of certain triggers including chocolate and cheese. Posture (particularly lying down) and straining (coughing and sneezing) are factors that worsen the headache of raised ICP. Drug use also causes headaches, for example use of glyceryl trinitrate, overuse of analgesics (rebound headache) and substance misuse or withdrawal.

Conversely, if simple analgesics such as paracetamol or ibuprofen have resolved the headache, it is unlikely that there is a serious underlying pathology. Rapidly progressive headache in the presence of neck stiffness, photophobia and fever should alert you to the possibility of acute meningitis.

Nature

Localising the headache can point to a cause: for example occipital (subarachnoid haemorrhage), eye pain (cluster headaches), unilateral and throbbing (migraine) or temporal with tender blood vessels (temporal arteritis). A tight band around the head is suggestive of a tension headache.

Associations

Associated symptoms and signs are shown in Table 5.1, which summarises common causes of headache.

Examination

All examinations should follow the airway, breathing, circulation, disability and exposure (ABCDE) approach (Resuscitation Council UK 2006). Patients with serious intracranial pathology, such as subarachnoid haemorrhage or raised ICP, may be critically unwell, requiring immediate emergency interventions. If the patient is unconscious, then airway, breathing and circulation support are the priority. In this case, neurological examination will usually reveal focal neurological signs, pupil abnormalities and heart rhythm and blood pressure abnormalities. Therefore, measurement of vital signs is of paramount importance. Indeed, the presence of a high fever would raise the suspicion of meningitis.

An examination should be performed to assess the conscious level, using the Glasgow Coma Scale (GCS; Jennet & Teasdale 1974) or the Alert, Voice, Pain, Unresponsive scale (American College of Surgeons 2003). A general examination should also be carried out and should include skin examination (non-blanching rash of meningococcal meningitis and bruising to suggest trauma), palpation (tender temporal arteries/pain on opening jaw in temporal arteritis) and assessment of neck stiffness. A full neurological examination will elicit any localising weakness or loss of sensation, for example in identifying the site of an SOL. Also, temporary weakness or loss of function may occur rarely with migraine. Visual assessment including visual acuity, visual fields (area of vision) and fundoscopy (looking in the back of the eyes) is important in helping to diagnose contralateral brain lesions (on the side opposite to the symptom) and papilloedema (swollen optic discs with blurred disc margins) from raised ICP.

While a headache is commonly a benign disorder, it is important that you are able to detect those with a more serious pathology. This is possible through good history and examination skills, following the TINA approach. If a serious intracranial pathology is considered, then a computed tomography (CT) scan is often required as the first line of imaging. However in the case of meningitis, this should not delay giving antibiotics.

Investigations

Vital signs: blood pressure, respiratory rate, oxygen saturations, temperature and heart rate.

White blood cell count, erythrocyte sedimentation rate (ESR), C-reactive protein (CRP) and blood cultures: to look for markers of infection in meningitis. The ESR is raised in temporal arteritis.

CT scan of the head: imaging of the brain will reveal haemorrhage, SOLs, swelling of the brain (cerebral oedema) and raised ICP. Magnetic resonance imaging (MRI) is used if CT is unable to reveal the cause (Figure 5.1).

Lumbar puncture: sampling of cerebrospinal fluid (CSF) that surrounds the brain and the spinal cord. CSF should be examined for abnormal protein and glucose levels and raised white blood cell count (bacterial and viral meningitis). Raised red blood cell count and blood-pigmented CSF (xanthochromia) occur with subarachnoid haemorrhage.

SYNCOPE

Syncope describes a temporary, self-limiting impairment of the conscious level, caused by a reduction in cerebral blood flow

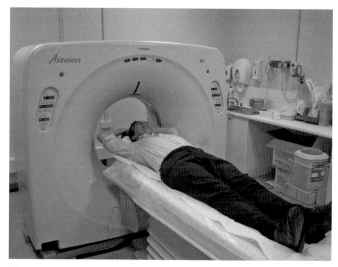

Figure 5.1 Computerise tomography (CT) scanning. [note the picture is of a CT scanner not an MRI scanner].

(Ballinger & Patchett 2003). It excludes seizure and coma. Syncope is also referred to as a 'blackout'. Pre-syncope describes the feeling of light-headedness, as if about to black out.

Syncope is prevalent among the population (Morag & Brenner 2008) and accounts for up to 3% of emergency department visits and 6% of hospital admissions each year. Fifty per cent of the population may experience syncope during their lifetime.

Causes

Syncope is very common, and there are many causes. These are shown in Table 5.2.

Syncope results from a reduction in cerebral blood flow. Maintaining an adequate heart rate, blood pressure and cardiac output is vital to ensure effective cerebral blood flow. A reduced cerebral blood flow results in lack of oxygen supply to the brainstem, in particular the area that is responsible for the conscious level.

Table 5.2 Common causes of syncope.

Non-cardiac	Hypoglycaemia Posterior circulation (brainstem) TIA Psychological – hyperventilation from a panic attack Severe anaemia Hypoxia Breath holding in children

Cardiac	Vasovagal syncope:
	  situational (fright/pain),
	  micturition (when passing urine) and
	  cough.
	Orthostatic/postural hypotension (low blood pressure when standing):
	  hypovolaemia (low blood volume);
	  after prolonged bed rest;
	  autonomic failure (e.g. in the elderly/diabetics);
	  drug induced (antihypertensives).
	Cardiac arrhythmias:
	  ventricular tachycardia;
	  supraventricular tachycardia;
	  sick sinus syndrome (failure of impulse to pass correctly through heart, causing bradycardia – slow pulse).
	
	Stokes–Adams (complete heart block, i.e. atrial activity does not pass to the ventricles, resulting in bradycardia of 15–40 bpm, or temporary asystole, i.e. no pulse). In the elderly this is usually due to fibrosis and calcification of the conduction system. In younger patients, it may be due to ischaemic heart disease.
	
	Carotid sinus syndrome (carotid sinus in neck is very sensitive to pressure).
	
	Cardiac outflow obstruction (e.g., aortic stenosis, hypertrophic obstructive cardiomyopathy).

Vasovagal syncope results from a reduction in venous return to the heart due to vasodilation causing venous pooling. The heart, which will then have a minimal blood volume, contracts vigorously, thus stimulating the receptors in the left ventricle. Reflexes via the central nervous system lead to further vasodilation and occasionally severe bradycardia. The poor venous return and vasodilation result in reduced blood flow to the brain, resulting in temporary loss of consciousness.

History and clinical examination

A syncopal attack can be sudden with no warning, although there may be a history of light-headedness, nausea, sweating, yawning, loss of vision or loss of hearing immediately prior to the episode. Consciousness is normally regained within a couple of minutes, and recovery is rapid if the cause is a simple vasovagal or orthostatic hypotension.

Whenever possible, it is helpful to obtain an eyewitness account of the events leading up to, during and after an episode of syncope. It is important to enquire about the situation in which the event occurred: for example had they been standing for a prolonged period (orthostatic hypotension), or did they have a shock or experience pain (vasovagal)? A witness may report that the patient's colour drained prior to the syncope (pallor).

A key difference in patients experiencing cardiac arrhythmias is that sudden flushing of the face may follow the initial pallor. The patient may also experience palpitations preceding the syncope. In patients who experience orthostatic hypotension, a drug history is relevant and must be sought, particularly of those drugs which lower the blood pressure or the heart rate, such as anti-hypertensives, anti-arrhythmics and opiates. The past medical history may reveal the following:

- diabetes (hypoglycaemia or autonomic dysfunction causing low blood pressure),
- ischaemic heart disease,
- heart failure (arrhythmias) and
- carotid hypersensitivity.

It is important to distinguish syncope from a seizure, for reasons which include impact on lifestyle and employment and also for treatment. A good history is vital. In syncope there may be some jerking movements of the limbs (complex vasovagal faint), but these are usually brief; recovery is rapid, and incontinence of urine is extremely uncommon. In a seizure, however, there are more likely to be persistent jerking movements, incontinence of urine and post-seizure (post-ictal) drowsiness.

Carotid sinus syndrome, although rare, is most common in the elderly. They may experience syncope with only the slightest pressure around their neck, for example because of a shirt collar or while having their hair washed at the hairdresser. Exertional syncope is rarer but is experienced by patients with cardiac outflow obstruction (aortic stenosis, cardiomyopathy), as the cardiac anomaly prevents cardiac output increasing on demand.

Immediately after vasovagal syncope, the patient may appear pale and clammy, though consciousness rapidly returns to normal. Ongoing drowsiness may indicate a post-ictal state after a seizure.

Cardiovascular examination may reveal heart murmurs (aortic stenosis, cardiomyopathy) or pulse abnormality. The pulse can help with diagnosis, by assessing rate and rhythm. Irregularity (arrhythmias), bradycardia (vasovagal), tachycardia (supraventricular tachycardia/ventricular tachycardia), alternating tachybrady (sick sinus) and transient asystole or bradycardia (Stokes–Adams) are all possibilities.

A consecutive lying–standing blood pressure should be taken to see if there is any significant drop in the systolic blood pressure (>20 mmHg) when going from lying to standing, which represents postural hypotension. A low blood pressure while lying indicates shock (hypovolaemia, sepsis or cardiogenic), and a patient with this is usually tachycardic, with poor capillary refill time and low urine output. There may be evidence of fluid loss (burns, bleeding). A full neurological examination should be carried out, though this will usually be normal, as syncope by definition is a self-limiting event.

There are many diagnoses to be considered for syncope. A thorough history with an eyewitness account, a detailed examination and the occasional appropriate use of simple tests can aid a correct diagnosis.

Specific investigations

Vital signs: blood pressure, respiratory rate, oxygen saturations, temperature and heart rate.

Serum blood glucose: to look for hypoglycaemia.

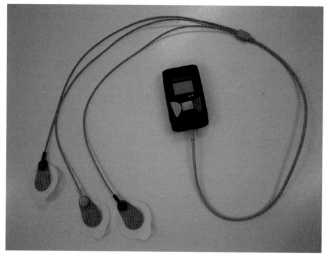

Figure 5.2 Twenty-four hour (Holter) ECG monitoring.

Full blood cell count: low haemoglobin in anaemia and raised white blood cell count in sepsis.

Urea and electrolytes: electrolyte abnormality such as high potassium (hyperkalaemia) may cause arrhythmias.

12-lead electrocardiogram (ECG): cardiac arrhythmias, cardiomyopathy.

24-h (Holter) ECG monitoring (Figure 5.2): identifies intermittent (paroxysmal) arrhythmias.

Echocardiogram: detailed scan of the heart for structural abnormalities such as valve stenosis and cardiomyopathy.

Electroencephalogram (EEG): to look at electrical activity in the brain, in difficult cases where syncope and seizure are indistinguishable.

Tilt-table testing: may aid the diagnosis of carotid hypersensitivity and postural hypotension. The patient is laid on a table which can be tilted to various angles and may provoke hypotension, bradycardia and syncope.

DIZZINESS

Dizziness is a very common symptom, and the word is used by patients to describe not only light-headedness but also vertigo, faintness, visual disturbance, confusion and loss of balance due to any cause. The most important distinction is between light-headedness (or presyncope, that is, the feeling that one is going to pass out) and true vertigo (which is the illusion of rotational movement, that is, the room spinning or the ground tilting).

Causes

The common causes of dizziness are shown in Table 5.3. The main differentiation is between acute and chronic permanent dizziness and multiple episodes of dizziness ('dizzy spells').

Light-headedness is often due to a reduction in cerebral blood perfusion that is not significant enough to cause loss of consciousness (syncope). The pathophysiology of vertigo is different however. The inner ear plays a vital role in both hearing and balance. The labyrinthine canals are concerned with balance, posture and movement, and therefore, anything that affects the middle ear may result in disruption of adequate control of these functions. Vertigo is the result of disease of the inner ear or the vestibulo-cochlear nerve (eighth cranial nerve).

History and clinical examination

Timing

The timing of an episode of dizziness may give a clue as to the cause, for example, dizziness after standing (postural hypotension), while breathing rapidly (hyperventilation) or on turning the head to one side (benign paroxysmal positional vertigo). The dizziness may develop after an ear infection, suggesting an upset in the inner ear (labyrinthitis or vestibular neuronitis).

Associated symptoms

Patients suffering with inner ear diseases, as a cause for their dizziness, may also report ringing in the ears (tinnitus) and deafness. This occurs in Meniere's disease where the patient experiences recurrent attacks of sudden-onset vertigo, tinnitus and progressive deafness. Less commonly, nausea, vomiting

Table 5.3 Common causes of dizziness.

	Differential diagnosis	Explanation
Permanent dizziness		
Acute onset	Labyrinthitis	Middle and inner ear inflammation
	Vestibular neuronitis	Inflammation of the vestibular nerve/labyrinth, causing severe vertigo and nystagmus
	Posterior circulation stroke	Stoke affecting the vertebro-basilar system, resulting in vertigo
Gradual onset	Cerebello-pontine angle tumour	Tumour of the eighth cranial nerve: an acoustic neuroma
	Ototoxicity	Drugs affect the ear system and thus balance and hearing, e.g. gentamicin and furosemide
	Multiple sclerosis	Affects predominantly the cerebellum and brainstem
Episodic dizziness		
	Meniere's disease	Attacks of vertigo, caused by increased pressure in the labyrinth; cause unknown
	Benign paroxysmal positional vertigo	Vertigo caused by certain head postures; likely to be due to vertebral artery ischaemia
	Recurrent posterior circulation TIAs	TIAs affecting the vertebra-basilar system, resulting in episodic dizziness
	Postural hypotension	Low blood pressure on sitting or standing, often due to hypertensive medication
	Hyperventilation and anxiety	Low circulating carbon dioxide levels resulting in dizziness

and photophobia could point towards migraine as an underlying cause. The sudden-onset dizziness associated with posterior circulation transient ischaemic attacks (TIAs) is due to ischaemia (insufficient cerebral blood flow) and may be associated with other neurological symptoms including facial muscle weakness, altered speech or vision and altered consciousness. To diagnose a TIA, all of the symptoms must have fully resolved within 24 h of onset.

Dizziness can be secondary to hyperventilation where a patient may report feeling anxious, rapid breathing and a tingling sensation around their mouth and in their fingers and toes. Taking slow deep breaths would resolve the symptoms in this case.

Palpitations would point to either an arrhythmia or an anxiety state being the cause of the dizziness. In multiple sclerosis, a chronic progressive disease affecting any part of the nervous system, there may also be limb weakness, poor vision, ataxia and dysarthria. Gradual onset of symptoms with associated deafness, numbness and paralysis of the face would make a diagnosis of a cerebello-pontine angle tumour more likely. A drug history should always be taken, in particular looking for drugs that may be causing damage to the ear (ototoxicity): gentamicin and furosemide are commonly found in clinical usage.

Examination

A thorough neurological examination is most helpful for guiding the clinician to a diagnosis. Assessment of hearing, balance and the eyes (for nystagmus, namely rapid involuntary movement of the eyes, which may be horizontal, vertical or rotational) will provide most of the information. Hearing can be informally assessed by talking to the patient both at a normal volume and by whispering.

Formal assessment is with the Rinne and Weber tests using a 512-Hz tuning fork. In the Rinne test, bone conduction is compared against air conduction. The vibrating tuning fork is placed just in front of the ear (air conduction) and then held against the mastoid bone behind the ear. Air conduction is normally better than bone conduction. The Weber test is performed by holding the vibrating tuning fork against the centre of the forehead. The sound should be heard equally in both ears.

Table 5.4 Comparing the Rinne and Weber tests in diagnosing deafness.

Deafness	Rinne test	Weber test
Sensorineural	AC > BC	Heard better in the good ear
Conductive	BC > AC	Heard better in the bad ear

BC, bone conduction; AC, air conduction.

Abnormalities of the inner ear are called sensorineural deafness, and these can be differentiated from conductive causes of deafness, such as earwax and middle ear infection, by combining the two tests (see Table 5.4).

Formal assessment of cranial nerves should be carried out looking at visual fields which may be affected in posterior circulation strokes and multiple sclerosis. Facial symmetry for facial palsies (weakness) and facial sensation should be examined, as abnormalities may also be indicative of TIAs, strokes or multiple sclerosis.

Fundoscopy in a patient with multiple sclerosis may reveal pale atrophied optic discs. Cerebellar disease may produce ataxia, an intention tremor (shaking of the hand when the arm is outstretched), nystagmus, incoordination, dysdiadochokinesia and dysarthria. Horizontal nystagmus occurs with ipsilateral (same-side) cerebellar disease and also with contralateral (opposite-side) vestibular disease, for example Meniere's disease and labyrinthitis. It is also necessary to perform a basic general examination, including pulse (arrhythmia), lying and standing blood pressure (postural hypotension) and auscultation of the heart for murmurs.

Dizziness is another presentation where a diagnosis can usually be made on the basis of the history and examination. Many of the associated features, for example tinnitus, hearing loss and nystagmus, can be very debilitating and unpleasant for the patient, even though they are not usually signs of a serious illness.

Specific investigations

Vital signs: blood pressure, respiratory rate, oxygen saturations, temperature and heart rate.

Lying and standing blood pressure.

Serum blood glucose: to look for hypoglycaemia.

Full blood cell count: low haemoglobin in anaemia.

Urea and electrolytes: electrolyte abnormality such as high potassium (hyperkalaemia) may cause arrhythmias.

12-lead ECG: to identify atrial fibrillation, other cardiac arrhythmias and valve disease.

24-h (Holter) ECG monitoring: identifies intermittent (paroxysmal) arrhythmias.

Audiometry: a detailed hearing test to assess the severity of hearing loss.

CT head: to identify areas of ischaemia and haemorrhage in stroke disease

MRI: to detect acoustic neuromas and identify areas of demyelination (destruction of the sheath surrounding nerve fibres) in multiple sclerosis.

Carotid Doppler ultrasound: to detect narrowed carotid arteries due to atherosclerosis.

Hallpike test: used to assess vertigo in benign paroxysmal positional vertigo. Patient lies flat on a couch, and the head is quickly and passively turned to one side. On turning the head the patient will experience vertigo and after a few seconds will also develop nystagmus which lessens on repeated testing.

Tilt-table testing: may aid the diagnosis of postural hypotension. The patient is laid on a table which can be tilted to various angles and may provoke hypotension, bradycardia and syncope.

SEIZURE

A seizure describes a temporary abnormal event resulting from a sudden electrical discharge from the cerebral nerves. A fit describes a 'sudden attack' (Martin 2010) and can be applied to any situation that is not necessarily neurological, for example a fit of coughing. A convulsion describes the involuntary contraction of muscles, producing contortion of the limbs or the torso (Martin 2010). Epilepsy is the tendency to recurrent seizure activity.

Incidence

Epilepsy is very common with 2% of the UK population having two or more seizures in their lifetime and 0.5% of the population having active epilepsy. However, in over 75% of patients who have isolated seizures, no cause is identified (Kumar & Clark 2005).

Causes

There are many causes of seizures, and these are shown in Table 5.5.

Normally, electrical activity in the brain is synchronised and restricted, resulting in limited neuronal discharges. In a seizure, this pattern becomes chaotic, and large groups of neurons are activated repetitively with failure of inhibition (stopping) of the disordered contact between the neurons. The pattern of

Table 5.5   Causes of seizures.

Neurological	Epilepsy Febrile convulsion – seizure associated with a fever, typically in infants and up to 6 years
Traumatic	Head injury Post-cranial surgery
Metabolic	Electrolyte abnormalities: hypernatraemia/hyponatraemia, hyperkalaemia/hypokalaemia, hypercalcaemia/hypocalcaemia Hypoxia (anoxic seizure) Hypoglycaemia Uraemia (high serum urea in renal failure)
Vascular	Subarachnoid haemorrhage Intracerebral haemorrhage Cerebral stroke
Infective	Bacterial meningitis Encephalitis Cerebral abscess
Neoplastic	Cerebral tumour
Drug induced	Alcohol excess/withdrawal Drug overdose/withdrawal, e.g. amphetamines, antipsychotics
Other	Pseudoseizures – non-epileptic seizures with a psychogenic basis

movements in a seizure is described as the tonic (increased tone, stiffness, no movement) and clonic (jerking, rhythmical movements) phases. In the tonic phase the patient may fall to the ground, clench their jaw, become cyanosed around the lips and face and hold their limbs in a fixed position. This is followed by the clonic phase where there may be rhythmical jerking of the limbs, tongue biting and urinary incontinence.

Seizures may be classified broadly into generalised and partial. A generalised seizure is one in which the abnormal electrical activity in the brain is widespread and the conscious level is always impaired. The most commonly recognised ones are as follows:

- tonic–clonic (grand mal),
- tonic,
- absence and
- myoclonic.

In a partial seizure, the abnormal electrical activity affects only a certain part of the brain, and the conscious level may not be impaired. These seizures may become generalised. Examples are as follows:

- simple partial,
- complex partial and
- partial with secondary generalisation.

History and clinical examination
This is another time when an eyewitness account of the event is invaluable. The information obtained should include the following:

- Colour of the patient – pallor (must exclude a complex vaso-vagal in which limb jerking can occur).
- Warning signs – the patient may describe that they did not feel quite right prior to the seizure:
  (1) prodrome – altered mood or behaviour;
  (2) aura – sensations, for example abnormal smell (temporal lobe epilepsy), visual disturbance and déjà vu.
- Abnormal behaviour – short vacant episodes, eyelids twitching and then returning to normal activity, apparently unaware

of the episode. This pattern is suggestive of a typical absence seizure.

- Description of the seizure – duration, progression, any altered conscious level, limb or body movements, incontinence and tongue biting.
- How the patient was afterwards – post-ictal phase (drowsiness) is common; if rapid resolution, consider vasovagal episode.
- Provoking factors:
  (1) concurrent illness – bacterial meningitis and febrile convulsion;
  (2) alcohol and drugs;
  (3) history of head injury;
  (4) lack of sleep;
  (5) flashing lights – a known trigger of epilepsy;
  (6) severe diarrhoea and vomiting – electrolyte disturbance.
- Past medical history and drug history:
  (1) known epileptic – always check drug compliance;
  (2) previous febrile convulsions;
  (3) SOL – brain tumour/abscess (previous tuberculosis);
  (4) previous TIAs and stroke;
  (5) renal failure;
  (6) diabetes.
- Family history: approximately 80% of patients with epilepsy have a first-degree relative with epilepsy.
- Associated symptoms:
  (1) Seizures with headache may be due to the following:
      head injury;
      meningitis (photophobia, pyrexia, neck stiffness, rash);
      SOL (headache worse in morning/on coughing, gradual onset, visual disturbance, vomiting, personality change);
      subarachnoid haemorrhage (sudden-onset, severe headache).
  (2) Other neurology:
      stroke (unilateral weakness, loss of speech);
      SOL (gradual progression of neurological symptoms).

A general examination may reveal the following:

- temperature – infective cause, febrile convulsion;
- signs of head injury;
- any injuries sustained during seizure;
- evidence of drug/alcohol abuse (aroma, needlestick marks);
- skin examination – rash, bruising.

A neurological examination should be performed to identify residual signs following the seizure. A normal post-ictal
period with reduced conscious level and generalised hypoto-
nia should be expected, but if the GCS remains low for a prolonged period, a metabolic cause or intracranial haemorrhage
should be considered. Pupil examination may reveal evidence
of drug use (pinpoint pupils in opiate use and dilated pupils
in amphetamine, ecstasy or benzodiazepine use). Non-reactive
dilated pupils may indicate raised ICP, and the fundi should
be examined for papilloedema. Cranial and peripheral nerve
examination should be carried out to look for limb and facial
weakness or altered sensation. Any residual neurological features usually warrants a CT scan of the head to exclude SOL or
intracranial haemorrhage.

Arriving at the correct differential diagnosis of a seizure can
prove difficult, and frequently no cause is identified, even with
the aid of specific investigations. The eyewitness account is particularly important, as it can exclude other simpler explanations
such as a vasovagal episode. It is important not to label a patient
with epilepsy without good supporting evidence, and epilepsy
should never be diagnosed after just one seizure.

Specific investigations

Vital signs: blood pressure, respiratory rate, oxygen saturations, temperature and heart rate.

Serum blood glucose: to look for hypoglycaemia.

Full blood cell count: raised white blood cell count in bacterial
meningitis or cerebral abscess.

Urea and electrolytes: hyperkalaemia/hypokalaemia, hyper-
natraemia/hyponatraemia and uraemia.

Serum calcium level: may reveal hypercalcaemia/
hypocalcaemia.

Arterial blood gases: may reveal hypoxia.

Blood cultures: should be taken prior to giving antibiotics if meningitis is suspected.

Urine/blood toxicology: drug screening.

Head CT scan: will reveal intracranial haemorrhage or SOL.

Lumbar puncture is essential if the diagnosis of meningitis or encephalitis is suspected.

EEG: to look for epileptiform activity in the brain and in difficult cases where syncope and seizure are indistinguishable.

TREMOR

A tremor is a rhythmical and alternating movement that may affect any part of the body (Martin 2010). It is the result of alternating contraction and relaxation of groups of muscles. All humans have a physiological tremor that is part of the normal mechanism for maintaining posture, although it may not be apparent at rest. It may become more pronounced when anxious or tired or after exercise.

Causes

There are three main groups of causes of tremor. The differential diagnosis is shown in Table 5.6.

History and clinical examination

Ask the patient to describe the tremor to you. This will aid classification initially. For example, a resting tremor is present in the arms at rest and is usually worse on one side. The tremor usually disappears when the patient makes voluntary movements. It frequently surrounds the small joints of the hand and is often described as a 'pill rolling' tremor. Other symptoms of parkinsonism include difficulty initiating walking, a slow and shuffling gait, generalised muscular rigidity and an expressionless face. An intention tremor occurs on movement, for example when reaching for a cup of tea. It is typically a coarse tremor. There may be a history of poor coordination, for example on brushing the hair and tying shoelaces, and difficulty with balance and speech difficulties. These are all symptoms of

Table 5.6 The differential diagnosis of tremor.

Type of tremor	Differential diagnosis
Resting tremor	Parkinsonism
Intention tremor	Cerebellar disease
Postural tremor	Essential tremor
Idiopathic	Anxiety, fatigue, exercise
Physiological	Hyperthyroidism
Pathological	Drugs
	Caffeine
	Alcohol
	Sodium valproate
	Lithium
	Beta agonists (e.g. salbutamol).
	Metabolic
	Carbon dioxide retention, e.g. COPD, asthma
	Hepatic encephalopathy
	Wilson's disease

cerebellar disease. A postural tremor also typically occurs on movement but is seen as a fine tremor of the hands.

The following details may lead to an underlying cause:

- A detailed drug and alcohol history must be taken to include the amount of caffeine consumed.
- A history of epilepsy should raise the possibility of drug-induced tremor.
- A history of asthma may point to the use of beta agonists.
- Family history may reveal that a number of relatives experience a tremor that disappears when supporting the limb. This is typical of a benign essential tremor. There are no other associated symptoms, and the patient may report that the tremor improves on taking alcohol.
- Symptoms including weight loss, heat intolerance, palpitations and diarrhoea point towards hyperthyroidism.
- If the tremor occurs only in certain situations, for example when angry or anxious, this suggests a physiological tremor.
- A history of liver disease, associated with altered mood or conscious level, may indicate hepatic encephalopathy.

- Wilson's disease is a rare metabolic disorder which results in copper being deposited in the liver and brain. Neurological symptoms including tremor, dementia and speech difficulties often appear in young adults.

A general examination should be carried out to look for signs of hyperthyroidism (tachycardia, atrial fibrillation, palmar erythema, thin hair, goitre and ophthalmoplegia), chronic liver disease (hepatomegaly, palmar erythema, spider naevi, ascites and clubbing) and respiratory disease (cyanosis, tachycardia, bounding pulse and chronic obstructive pulmonary disease [COPD]). Rarely, Wilson's disease is revealed by the presence of a Kayser–Fleischer copper-coloured ring around the cornea.

Cerebellar function should be examined to look for the following:

- nystagmus;
- dysarthria;
- reduced muscle tone;
- diminished reflexes;
- incoordination when performing rapid alternating movement (dysdiadochokinesia) and
- impaired coordination of repetitive heel–shin test.

A gait examination is mandatory to look for the following:

- Ataxic gait – wide-based, unsteady and unable to walk heel-to-toe along a straight line. This is a feature of cerebellar disease.
- Shuffling gait – stooped posture, difficulty initiating movement, slow, shuffling and with minimal arm swing. This is a feature of parkinsonism. Also look for an expressionless face, rigidity of limbs, monotonous speech and drooling.

Assessment of the tremor should be undertaken. Look at the upper limbs at rest to determine whether any tremor is present. If so, it is likely to be that of parkinsonism. Look for the coarse action that resembles someone rolling a pill between their thumb and fingers. When this patient becomes involved in active movement, the tremor is likely to improve.

Ask the patient to stretch out their hands and to touch your finger held an arm's breadth in front of them. If the tremor appears here, it is likely to be an intention tremor or a postural tremor. If the tremor can be overcome by supporting the arm, benign essential tremor is the likely diagnosis (it may be helpful to place a piece of paper on the outstretched hands to demonstrate a fine tremor). An intention tremor becomes more pronounced when the patient's finger approaches that of the examiner. Often the patient will not in fact be able to fully control the movement and will therefore point past the examiner's finger. Postural tremors are often coarser and become more obvious on posturing to hold a cup or pick up a piece of paper.

A detailed history of the tremor must be taken to reach the correct diagnosis. History and examination will reveal whether the tremor is resting, intention or postural, and a general examination should be undertaken to look for systemic causes. Clinical diagnosis is usually possible, and only simple tests are required.

Specific investigations

Vital signs: blood pressure, respiratory rate, oxygen saturations, temperature and heart rate.

Thyroid function tests: to look for hyperthyroidism.

Liver function tests: to look for features of chronic liver disease.

Arterial blood gases: to look for carbon dioxide retention.

Serum levels: of sodium valproate or lithium.

MRI head scan: for assessment of cerebellar disease.

HEMIPLEGIA

Hemiplegia is total paralysis of one side of the body (Martin 2010). Hemiparesis describes weakness of one side of the body and includes hemiplegia.

A hemiplegia is usually the result of a cerebral hemisphere lesion on the side opposite (contralateral) to the paralysis. The most common cause is damage to the cerebral neurons by ischaemic stroke, but other causes are prevalent (as described later). Motor weakness is usually (but not always) accompanied by sensory loss in the same distribution, because of the

Table 5.7 Causes of hemiplegia.

Cause	Differential diagnosis
Vascular	Ischaemic stroke or TIA
	High spinal infarction due to spinal artery thrombosis
	Intracerebral haemorrhage
	Cerebral vasculitis
Traumatic	Subdural haematoma
	Extradural haematoma
Other	Multiple sclerosis
	Cerebral tumour
	Cerebral abscess
	Epilepsy (transient hemiplegia)
	Migraine (transient hemiplegia)

proximity of the motor and sensory cortices in the brain. The lesion is always within the central nervous system. Indeed, peripheral neuropathies cause local nerve damage, leading to localised muscle weakness and loss of sensation only.

Causes

Hemiplegia is frequently caused by a sudden cerebral event, such as an ischaemic stroke or a haemorrhage. A more insidious onset suggests a different pathology. The causes of hemiplegia are shown in Table 5.7.

History and clinical examination

The history of a hemiplegia is most likely to be obtained from a relative, friend or carer. Determine the speed at which hemiplegia occurred. Hemiplegia of rapid onset is most likely to be due to a sudden cerebral event, for example a transient ischaemic attack (TIA), an ischaemic stroke or a haemorrhage. Hemiplegia that gradually develops is usually due to an insidious problem, such as an SOL, a chronic subdural haemorrhage or multiple sclerosis, where gradual demyelination results in slow progression of neurological symptoms. A past medical history may reveal some of the many risk factors for stroke disease, including atrial fibrillation, hypertension, diabetes, ischaemic heart disease, smoking, hypercholesterolaemia, previous strokes, clotting abnormalities and alcoholism. A patient who has had a recent infective illness, particularly of the middle ear or the sinus, or an infection associated with foreign travel may have a cerebral abscess from local or blood-borne spread. Anticoagulated patients are at risk of intracranial haemorrhage.

A TIA, an ischaemic stroke or an intracerebral haemorrhage can present with a hemiparesis if the motor cortex is affected by the lesion. The face and arms are often affected more than the leg, and weakness is more profound in these muscle groups. However, strokes affecting the anterior cerebral circulation produce hemiparesis affecting the leg more than the arms. Additionally, if other areas of the cerebral cortex are affected, the patient will present with corresponding features, such as visual loss, auditory loss, speech disturbance and personality change. A patient who has presented with a hemiplegia following a seizure may have an epileptic hemiplegia (Todd's paresis). If the hemiplegia resolves quickly, this is likely to be the case. However, it is dangerous to assume this initially, as continuing features may represent a more serious underlying pathology. If the hemiplegia is associated with a headache, usually with a prior history of headaches, the possibility of hemiplegic migraine is raised; once again the hemiplegia is transient. A recent history of head injury suggests an extradural or a subdural haemorrhage, and the hemiplegia may develop over hours to days. However the injury may be trivial, particularly in alcohol abusers and elderly patients. Gradual-onset hemiplegia may be associated with a number of other features associated with raised ICP, if the headache is due to an SOL. This might include morning headaches, loss of vision, vomiting and altered conscious level. Multiple sclerosis is a chronic and often relapsing and remitting disease, in which the patient experiences intermittent episodes of altered neurological function, due to damage to the myelin sheath surrounding any neuron in the central nervous system. Therefore other features may include weakness, ataxia, nystagmus, double vision, dysarthria and altered sensation. The patient may report similar previous episodes.

Cardiovascular examination may give some clues to possible causes. The pulse may be irregular (atrial fibrillation causes

Table 5.8 Clinical syndromes associated with a variety of central nervous system lesions.

Site of lesion	Clinical syndrome
Brainstem (commonly stroke, tumour or multiple sclerosis)	Reduced conscious level Hemiplegia Ipsilateral facial weakness Contralateral arm and leg weakness
Middle cerebral artery territory (parieto-temporal lobe – any cause)	Hemiplegia Hemisensory loss Contralateral facial weakness Visual disturbance, dysphasia, apraxia or confusion
Anterior cerebral artery territory (frontal lobe – any cause)	Hemiplegia Intellectual impairment Visual disturbance Dysphasia Personality change

embolic stroke). Splinter haemorrhages, palmar vascular lesions, clubbing and new heart murmurs may represent infective endocarditis, which can result in ischaemic or septic emboli and thus cerebral stroke or abscess respectively. Carotid bruits may be heard in the presence of carotid atherosclerosis. Complete neurological examination, including the GCS score, cranial nerves, peripheral nervous system and cerebellum, will provide the most information in identifying both the cause and the site of a central nervous system lesion. A variety of clinical syndromes and the corresponding lesion sites are shown in Table 5.8.

Neurological examination will reveal a hemiplegia, and additional features may point to a lesion site within the central nervous system. History and general examination will lead to a likely underlying cause. However, imaging of the brain is almost always required to make a formal diagnosis and determine the nature of an SOL.

Specific investigations

Vital signs: blood pressure, respiratory rate, oxygen saturations, temperature and heart rate.

White blood cell count, ESR, CRP and blood cultures: to look for markers of infection in cerebral abscess; white blood cells may be raised in ischaemic stroke.

Clotting screen: to look for clotting abnormalities.

Serum calcium: often increased in disseminated malignancy.

Serum lipids: a risk factor for stroke.

12-lead ECG: will show atrial fibrillation.

Chest X-ray: may show a focus of infection.

CT head scan: will reveal the site of haemorrhage, ischaemic stroke, skull fracture, tumour or abscess.

MRI scan (head and spine): SOL, areas of focal demyelination and plaques associated with multiple sclerosis.

Lumbar puncture: fluid for electrophoresis to identify oligoclonal bands and paraproteins associated with multiple sclerosis.

Electroencephalogram (EEG): may show epileptiform activity.

Carotid Doppler ultrasound: to reveal carotid artery stenosis in stroke disease.

ACUTE CONFUSION

Acute confusion describes a state of altered consciousness in which mental clarity and reasoning are impaired. Impairment of attention and memory and abnormal perception such as visual hallucinations are seen, and the condition classically fluctuates over time. Confusion is an acute presentation in which fluctuating conscious level is often seen, whereas dementia is a slow decline in cognitive function over a number of months or years, and the conscious level is unaffected.

Acute confusion is seen in a large minority of hospital inpatients, and up to 20% of acutely ill hospital inpatients. A brain already in decline predisposes to further impairment, so confusion is most often seen in elderly patients who already have dementia.

Causes

A large number of diseases cause confusion, but some of the more common ones are shown in Table 5.9. Causes of dementia are not considered.

Table 5.9 Common causes of confusion.

Metabolic	Hypoglycaemia
	Hyponatraemia
	Renal failure
	Liver failure
	Hypercalcaemia
	Hyperthyroidism/hypothyroidism
Infection	Urinary tract infection
	Pneumonia
	Meningo-encephalitis
	Sepsis syndrome (from any other cause)
Neurological	Subdural haemorrhage
	Intracerebral haemorrhage
	Ischaemic stroke or TIA
	Epilepsy (temporal lobe, post-ictal phase)
	Cerebral tumour
Drugs	Alcohol or drug intoxication or withdrawal
	Opiate use or misuse
	Anticonvulsants
	Drugs of abuse – cannabis, opiates, amphetamines
	Sedative drugs – benzodiazepines
Hypoxia	Respiratory disease – respiratory failure particularly in COPD and severe pneumonia
	Cardiac disease – cardiac failure, arrhythmia, myocardial infarction

History and clinical examination

There are a number of typical features of confusion which may be present:

- Reduced conscious level – fluctuant deterioration over hours or days, which is typically worse at night. The patient has a reduced awareness of their surroundings.
- Altered thinking – may be slow and muddled, with or without fixed, false beliefs (delusions).
- Disorientation – in time and place.
- Altered behaviour – abnormal for the patient, either hyperactivity and irritability or underactivity. The patient may be more withdrawn.

- Altered perception – illusions and hallucinations (often visual).
- Altered mood – fluctuating mood and affect.
- Poor memory (short and long terms) and recall.

A key part of taking the history is to establish whether confusion is new and acute, rather than part of a long-standing dementia syndrome. It will frequently be very difficult to obtain a history from the patients themselves, and therefore, relatives, carers or professionals in primary care will provide invaluable information.

- Onset of confusion
  (1) Sudden – likely to be hypoxia, a metabolic disorder or neurological disease.
  (2) A history of seizures or preceding fit suggests post-ictal phase in epilepsy.
  (3) A history of head injury suggests intracranial haemorrhage or brain injury. However, a subdural haemorrhage commonly presents subacutely with worsening confusion and only a trivial history of head injury.
  (4) Sudden onset with limb or facial weakness and altered sensation suggests stroke or TIA.
  (5) Subacute onset suggests a metabolic disorder such as thyroid disease or liver failure but also slow onset of neurological disease as in a cerebral tumour or abscess.
- Past medical history
  (1) Thyroid disease.
  (2) Diabetes – enquire about the patient's blood glucose control, medication compliance and intercurrent infection that may provoke deranged blood glucose.
  (3) Malignancy – risk of hypercalcaemia, cerebral metastases or immunosuppression causing infection.
  (4) Liver disease – alcohol use, viral hepatitis, drug history and malignancy.
  (5) History of alcohol intoxication and withdrawal.
  (6) Chronic kidney disease causing electrolyte disturbance and uraemia. The patient may have a history of hypertension, diabetes and recurrent urinary infections.

- Drug history
  (1) The patient may reveal a history of illicit drug or alcohol use.
  (2) Ask about accidental overdose of prescribed medication.
  (3) Use of opiate analgesia.
  (4) Sedative drugs – benzodiazepines.
  (5) Cardiac drugs, diuretics and anti-hypertensive drugs may cause electrolyte disturbance.
  (6) Use of anticonvulsants, antidepressants, thyroid medication or inhalers can suggest underlying chronic disease.

A general examination may reveal the following:

- Smell of breath – alcohol or ketotic ('pear drops').
- Skin examination
  (1) Purpuric rash – meningo-encephalitis.
  (2) Needlestick tracks – illicit drug use and overdose.
  (3) Evidence of deliberate self-harm.
  (4) Bruising – trauma to skull, causing lacerations and haematomas; behind the ears (Battle's sign); surrounding eyes (racoon eyes).
  (5) Infection – open wounds, abscess or cellulitis.
- Evidence of underlying disease
  (1) Hyperthyroidism – anorexia, goitre and thin hair.
  (2) Hypothyroidism – dry skin and coarse facial features.
  (3) Liver disease – spider naevi, jaundice, ascites and palmar erythema.
  (4) Kidney disease – hypertension and pallor.
  (5) Respiratory – cyanosis.
  (6) Peripheral and central cyanosis – respiratory failure, cardiac failure, severe sepsis or myxoedema crisis.

Cardiac, respiratory and abdominal examinations are mandatory to look for signs of underlying chronic or metabolic disease or active infection. The neurological examination is important to look for focal signs that reveal an underlying neurological cause, and it also acts as a guide to the severity.

The neurological examination should include the following:

- an assessment of the conscious level (the GCS or the Alert, Voice, Pain, Unresponsive scale);

- pupil examination (size and reaction to light);
- cranial nerve examination;
- peripheral nervous system examination;
- examination of the patient's gait;
- a cerebellum examination.

The patient's cognitive function should be formally assessed using the Abbreviated Mental Test Score (AMTS), developed by Hodkinson in 1972 as a quick, valid method of determining the presence and severity of confusion in a number of domains. A score of less than 7 suggests abnormal cognitive function (Jitapunkul *et al*. 1991). The AMTS is shown in Table 5.10.

A patient with acute confusion is often difficult to assess, as cooperation with history taking and examination is often poor. Differentiation between chronic and acute confusion is helpful, but there is often overlap, as confusion most commonly occurs in those with poor cognitive function. Causes are many and varied, so a detailed history is important, and this is usually from

Table 5.10 The AMTS. Adapted from Hodkinson (1972).

Question	Score
What is your age?	0 or 1
What is the time (to the nearest hour)?	0 or 1
Give the patient an address, and ask them to repeat it at the end of the test, e.g. '42 West Street'. Ask the patient to repeat to ensure they have heard it.	
What is the year?	0 or 1
What is the name of the hospital or the number of the residence where the patient is situated?	0 or 1
Can the patient recognise two persons (the doctor, nurse, home help, etc.)?	0 or 1
What is your date of birth?	0 or 1
In which year did the First World War begin? (Adjust this for a world event the patient would have known during childhood.)	0 or 1
What is the name of the present monarch (or the head of state)? Count backwards from 20 to 1.	0 or 1
Repeat the address.	0 or 1
	Score /10

a relative or a carer; knowledge of the patient's previous diagnoses and drug history is essential. Detailed examination may reveal localising neurological features, but the diagnosis is usually made after a series of basic investigations.

Specific investigations

Vital signs: blood pressure, respiratory rate, oxygen saturations, temperature and heart rate.

Fingertip blood glucose: immediate measure of glycaemic control.

Random plasma glucose.

Urea and electrolytes: hyponatraemia and renal failure.

Liver function tests: to look for chronic liver disease or liver failure.

Serum calcium: may be raised.

Thyroid function tests: in hypothyroidism or hyperthyroidism.

Toxicology screen: blood for paracetamol and salicylate levels, and urine for metabolites of drugs of abuse.

Arterial blood gases: to look for type 2 respiratory failure.

White blood cell count, ESR, CRP and blood cultures: to look for markers of infection in cerebral infection or septicaemia.

Clotting screen: to look for clotting abnormalities in haemorrhage.

12-lead ECG: will show bradyarrhythmia and tachyarrhythmia.

Chest X-ray: may show a focus of infection.

CT head scan: will reveal the site of haemorrhage, skull fracture, tumour or abscess.

Lumbar puncture: sampling of CSF for abnormal protein and glucose levels and raised white blood cell count (bacterial and viral meningitis); raised red blood cell count and blood-pigmented CSF (xanthochromia) with small subarachnoid haemorrhages not seen on the CT scan.

Electroencephalogram (EEG): may show epileptiform activity.

REDUCED CONSCIOUS LEVEL AND COMA

Consciousness is a state of wakefulness and awareness, and reduced conscious level describes drowsiness with reduced awareness. The GCS was designed in 1974 by Jennet and Teasdale as a measure of reduced conscious level, using eye opening and verbal and motor responses as markers of consciousness. A low conscious level (GCS score of fewer than 9) is compatible with a coma.

Causes

There are a variety of causes of reduced conscious level and coma, and those commonly seen in clinical practice are shown in Table 5.11.

Table 5.11 Causes of reduced conscious level and coma.

Traumatic head injury	Subdural or extradural haemorrhage Subarachnoid haemorrhage Diffuse axonal injury
Cerebral	Seizure and post-ictal period SOL – tumour or abscess
Vascular	Ischaemic or haemorrhagic stroke Subarachnoid haemorrhage Hypertensive encephalopathy
Metabolic	Hypoglycaemia Diabetic ketoacidosis and hyperosmolar non-ketotic coma
	Hyponatraemia Hypothermia Addisonian crisis
Organ failure	Respiratory – hypoxia and hypercarbia Cardiac – hypotension due to cardiogenic shock, ruptured aneurysm, bradyarrhythmia or tachyarrhythmia
	Renal – uraemic encephalopathy Hypothyroidism – myxoedematous coma Hyperthyroidism – thyrotoxic storm
Infection	Meningo-encephalitis Septicaemia and septic shock Cerebral malaria
Toxins	Carbon monoxide poisoning Alcohol intoxication Drugs (tricyclic antidepressants, opiates, benzodiazepines) General anaesthesia

The area of the brain that is responsible for coordinating the conscious level is the brainstem reticular formation. Reduced conscious level is the result of a combination of three processes, which affect the brainstem reticular formation and the cerebral cortex:

(1) Diffuse brain dysfunction affecting all parts of the brain – caused by metabolic, toxic or neurological disorders.
(2) A direct effect on the brainstem – lesions within the brainstem, such as multiple sclerosis, ischaemic or haemorrhagic stroke or tumour, damage the reticular formation directly.
(3) Indirect pressure effect on the brainstem – cortical or cerebellar lesions that occupy space produce a pressure effect on the brainstem. Lesions such as cortical or cerebellar lesions and subdural haemorrhage that occupy space produce a pressure effect on the brainstem.

History and clinical examination

In a patient presenting with reduced conscious level, there may be limited or no history available, especially if the patient has been found alone. However, a collateral history should be sought from relatives, witnesses or the emergency services. It may be that the only information available is from primary care or previous hospital records. As a rule, if the conscious level is fluctuating with a gradual onset, the cause is likely to be metabolic, but in the case of brain injury after haemorrhage or head injury, there is usually a rapid one-way deterioration in the conscious level.

Any past medical history is of paramount importance, and a history of the following should be sought:

• Diabetes:
   (1) Diabetic ketoacidosis – type 1 diabetics, for example with concurrent illness/poor compliance (may be first presentation).
   (2) Hypoglycaemic coma – rapid onset, associated with sweating and preceding agitation.
   (3) Hyperosmolar non-ketosis – type 2 diabetics.

- Thyroid disease – recent surgery, radioiodine, infection or epilepsy.
- Respiratory – type 2 respiratory failure in COPD or asthma.
- Cardiac – ischaemic heart disease, arrhythmia or valve disease.
- Hypertension.
- Psychiatric disorder or history of drug/alcohol abuse.
- Chronic renal disease.
- Malignancy.
- Recent surgery – ear, nose and throat procedures/neurosurgery (cerebral abscess).

Accompanying features are important along with the history immediately preceding the current illness:

- Fever, night sweats, rash, sore throat, cough and lower urinary tract symptoms suggest infection.
- Headache, visual or speech disturbance and limb weakness or abnormal sensation suggest intracranial pathology.
- A seizure suggests post-ictal phase but may be due to an SOL or meningo-encephalitis.
- Low mood and abnormal behaviour – possible overdose.
- Chest pain, palpitation or breathlessness suggest cardiorespiratory disease.
- Vomiting is seen in the context of infection and raised ICP.
- Recent infection, trauma and surgery often act as precipitants for many of the metabolic causes of coma.
- Polydipsia, polyuria, lethargy and abdominal pain suggest diabetic ketoacidosis or hyperosmolar non-ketosis.
- A history of foreign travel to the tropics may suggest cerebral malaria.

A drug history may reveal the following:

- steroid use;
- medication used in a variety of cardiac, respiratory or metabolic diseases;
- drugs used in neurological disease, such as anti-epileptics;
- psychiatric drugs including sedatives;
- painkillers including opioids.

The external environment is important, and the following factors should be taken into account:

- empty medication bottles or suicide note – drug overdose;
- medic-alert bracelet – for example epilepsy or diabetes;
- needles and syringes – drug abuse;
- empty alcohol containers;
- evidence of trauma or history of injury – head injury;
- young people, late at night – alcohol intoxication or drug overdose;
- multiple house occupants – carbon monoxide poisoning.

In a patient presenting with coma, rapid assessment and management are the priorities. The initial assessment should use the ABCDE approach with immobilisation of the C-spine if there is any concern over injury. Prior to continuing a general examination, any airway, breathing or circulation compromise should be dealt with. Documentation of a baseline GCS and full neurological observations including pupil size and reaction, heart rate, blood pressure, temperature and respiratory rate is important so that any change is evident later on.

A general examination may reveal the following:

- Smell of breath – alcohol or ketotic ('pear drops').
- Skin examination
  - (1) Purpuric rash – meningo-encephalitis.
  - (2) Needlestick tracks – illicit drug use and overdose.
  - (3) Evidence of deliberate self-harm.
  - (4) Bruising – trauma to the skull, causing lacerations and haematomas; behind the ears (Battle's sign); surrounding the eyes (racoon eyes).
  - (5) Infection – open wounds, abscess or cellulitis.
- Evidence of underlying disease
  - (1) Hyperthyroidism – anorexia, goitre and thin hair.
  - (2) Hypothyroidism – dry skin and coarse facial features.
  - (3) Liver disease – spider naevi, jaundice, ascites and palmar erythema.
  - (4) Kidney disease – hypertension and pallor.
  - (5) Respiratory – cyanosis.
  - (6) Peripheral and central cyanosis – respiratory failure, cardiac failure, severe sepsis or myxoedema crisis.

Cardiac, respiratory and abdominal examinations are mandatory to look for signs of underlying chronic or metabolic disease or active infection. The neurological examination is important to look for focal signs that reveal an underlying neurological cause, and it also acts as a guide to the severity and subsequent prognosis.

Pupil examination (size and reaction to light) may reveal the following:

- Bilateral fixed, dilated pupils – sign of brain death by herniation of the brainstem or very deep coma (especially if induced by hypothermia or tricyclic overdose).
- Unilateral fixed, dilated pupil – coning (herniation) of the temporal lobe or compression of the third cranial nerve (oculomotor), for example by ipsilateral tumour or haemorrhage. This requires urgent neurosurgical opinion.
- Bilateral unreactive, pinpoint pupils – opiate overdose.
- Small pupils that react to light – metabolic-induced coma and brainstem lesions.
- Bilateral dilated pupils – benzodiazepines, cocaine or amphetamines.

Examination of the fundi may reveal papilloedema in the case of raised ICP or hypertensive encephalopathy. Fundoscopy may reveal evidence of retinal haemorrhage due to head trauma.

The remainder of the neurological examination is limited when a patient is in a coma but should include all parts of the cranial nerves and peripheral nervous system, paying particular attention to the symmetry of signs. Assessment of sensory loss is not possible in coma.

- Facial weakness.
- Assessment of tone in the limbs – increased or decreased.
- Assessment of limb movement, both active and passive.
- Reflexes – including Babinski (plantar); often extensor if the cause is related to the central nervous system.

Immediate assessment and management using the ABCDE approach is of utmost importance, as primarily the airway is at risk in a patient with reduced conscious level. Neurological examinations may reveal the site and severity of any intracranial lesion, but a variety of systematic and metabolic causes may not be easily recognisable without some basic investigations. However a past medical history of chronic disease or prescribed medication may point towards a diagnosis.

Specific investigations

Vital signs: blood pressure, respiratory rate, oxygen saturations, temperature and heart rate.

Fingertip blood glucose: immediate measure of glycaemic control.

Random plasma glucose.

Urea and electrolytes: hyponatraemia, Addisonian crisis or renal failure.

Liver function tests: to look for chronic liver disease.

Serum calcium: may be raised in malignancy.

Thyroid function tests: in hypothyroidism or hyperthyroidism.

Random cortisol: may be low in Addisonian crisis.

Toxicology screen: blood for paracetamol and salicylate levels, and urine for metabolites of drugs of abuse.

Arterial blood gases: to look for type 2 respiratory failure and the carboxyhaemoglobin level in carbon monoxide poisoning.

White blood cell count, ESR, CRP and blood cultures: to look for markers of infection in cerebral infection or septicaemia.

Clotting screen: to look for clotting abnormalities in haemorrhage.

12-lead ECG: will show bradyarrhythmia and tachyarrhythmia.

Chest X-ray: may show a focus of infection.

CT head scan: will reveal the site of haemorrhage, skull fracture, tumour or abscess.

Lumbar puncture: sampling of CSF for abnormal protein and glucose levels and raised white cell count (bacterial and viral meningitis); raised red blood cell count and blood-pigmented CSF (xanthochromia) with small subarachnoid haemorrhages not seen on the CT scan.

Electroencephalogram (EEG): may show epileptiform activity.

REFERENCES

American College of Surgeons. (2003) *Advanced Trauma Life Support Course Manual*, 8th edn. American College of Surgeons, Chicago.

Ballinger, A. & Patchett, S. (2003) *Pocket Essentials of Clinical Medicine*, 3rd edn. W. B. Saunders, Edinburgh, UK.

Hodkinson, H.M. (1972) Evaluation of a mental test score for assessment of mental impairment in the elderly. *Age and Ageing* **1**, 233–238.

Jennet, B. & Teasdale, G. (1974) Assessment of coma and impaired consciousness. A practical scale. *Lancet* **ii**, 81–83.

Jitapunkul, S., Pillay, I. & Ebrahim, S. (1991) The abbreviated mental test: its use and validity. *Age and Ageing* **20**, 332–336.

Kumar, P. & Clark, M. (2005) *Clinical Medicine*, 6th edn. W. B. Saunders, Edinburgh, UK.

Martin, A. (ed.) (2010) *Oxford Concise Medical Dictionary*, 8th edn. Oxford University Press, Oxford.

Morag, R. & Brenner, B.E. (2008) *Syncope*. E-medicine, WebMD. http://www.emedicine.com/emerg/topic876.htm

Resuscitation Council UK. (2006) *Advanced Life Support (ALS)*, 5th edn. Resuscitation Council UK, London.

6 Clinical Diagnosis of Symptoms Associated with the Musculoskeletal System

Michael Parry

The aim of this chapter is to understand the clinical diagnosis of symptoms associated with the musculoskeletal system.

LEARNING OUTCOMES
At the end of this chapter, the reader will be able to discuss the clinical diagnosis of the following symptoms associated with the neurological system:

❏ muscle wasting and weakness,
❏ painful joints,
❏ deformity and
❏ loss of function.

MUSCLE WASTING AND WEAKNESS
A muscle is defined as either voluntary or involuntary. An involuntary muscle is that which functions free of conscious control and is made up of the smooth muscle found in the gut and blood vessels and the cardiac muscle of the heart. A voluntary muscle, as the name implies, is under conscious control. This

Clinical Diagnosis, 1st edition. Edited by Phil Jevon.
© 2011 Blackwell Publishing Ltd.

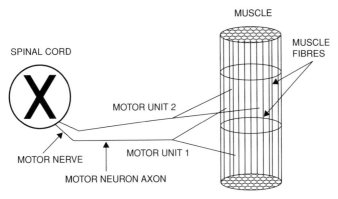

Figure 6.1 The motor unit comprising a motor nerve dividing to supply each individual muscle unit.

muscle constitutes the contractile muscle responsible for movement of joints and the muscles of facial expression.

The skeletal muscle has a structure of multiple repeating units of proteins that are able to very rapidly bind to and unbind from each other, allowing each protein unit to slide over its neighbour and therefore reduce in length. Each muscle group (for example the biceps) receives a nervous input from a single motor nerve which divides to supply each individual muscle unit.

Therefore, as shown from Figure 6.1, muscle wasting can result from a disorder at any one of these stages: the brain, the spinal cord, the motor nerve or the muscle unit itself.

Causes of muscle wasting
A muscle is a dynamic structure that requires constant input to remain functional. The causes of muscle wasting are shown next.

Neurogenic causes of muscle wasting
- Disorders affecting the brain: following a stroke, space-occupying lesion (for example a tumour) or head injury.
- Disorders affecting the spinal cord: spinal cord compression caused by a fracture, as seen in Figures 6.2 and 6.3, tumour, abscess, disc, as seen in Figure 6.4, and vertebral lesions,

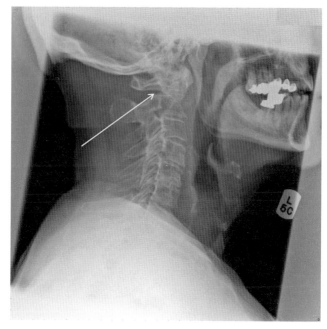

Figure 6.2 Plain lateral radiographs of acute cervical spinal injuries.

epidural haemorrhage or syringomyelia (a fluid-filled cavity within the spinal cord).
- Degenerative neuronal diseases: motor neuron disease or spinal muscular atrophy.
- Polyneuropathies: systemic conditions affecting multiple nerves, which may be toxic or metabolic and caused by drugs or vitamin deficiencies; for example Guillain–Barre syndrome, hereditary sensorimotor neuropathy, autoimmune neuropathy and polyneuropathy in cancer.
- Mononeuropathies: peripheral nerve compression or entrapment (for example carpal tunnel syndrome, meralgia paraesthetica) or traumatic nerve injury.
- Neuromuscular junction disorders: diseases affecting the transmission of signal from the nerve end plate to the muscle

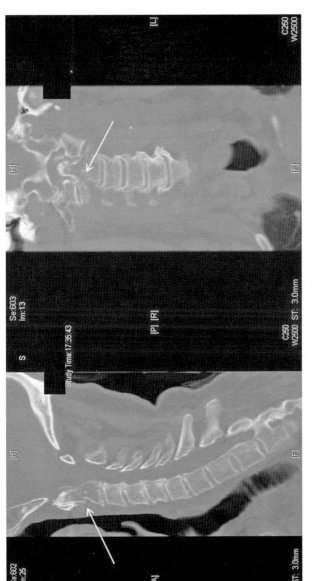

Figure 6.3 CT scan of the same neck injury, showing fracture through the odontoid peg (arrows).

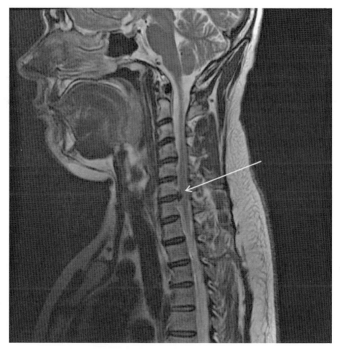

Figure 6.4   Central disc protrusion seen on MRI at the C6/C7 level.

fibre; for example myasthenia gravis (antibodies to the acetyl-choline receptor, causing interference and destruction of the receptor).

Non-neurogenic causes of muscle wasting

- Inflammatory myopathies: inflammatory conditions of skeletal muscles, causing pain and weakness.
- Metabolic and endocrine myopathies: such as proximal muscle weakness caused by corticosteroids in high doses and other conditions due to thyroid disease, drugs, alcohol excess and calcium deficiency.
- Muscular dystrophies: progressive genetically determined conditions affecting the skeletal muscle (for example

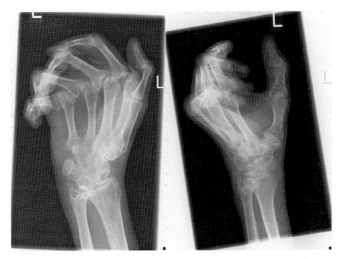

Figure 6.5 Typical X-ray features of rheumatoid arthritis seen in the hands.

Duchenne muscular dystrophy, facioscapulohumeral dystrophy).

- Disuse atrophy: reduction in muscle mass and therefore weakness due to disuse of the muscle (for example in astronauts and because of prolonged bed rest and immobilisation in a cast).

History and clinical examination
Muscle atrophy should be differentiated from the progressive muscle wasting of sarcopaenia seen in old age and cachexia seen in conditions such as cancer and HIV and following burn injuries.

A full history and examination should first be undertaken. From the history, details such as trauma, the progression of the symptoms and associated drug or alcohol use should be noted. A full neurological examination and examination of the pertinent joint will often identify the cause of the wasting or weakness. Specific investigations are aimed at identifying the cause of the wasting.

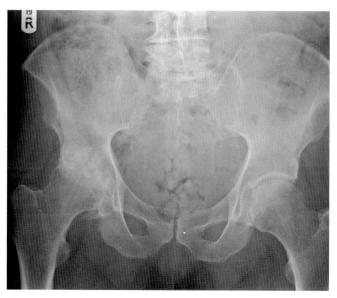

Figure 6.6 X-ray of the hips, showing the characteristic features of osteoarthritis in the right hip: joint space narrowing, subchondral sclerosis, osteophyte formation and subchondral cyst formation.

Specific investigations

Blood tests

- Full blood count and film: anaemia of chronic disease in polyneuropathies and malignancy, raised white blood cell count in infectious causes of weakness (for example spinal or intracranial abscess), raised mean corpuscular volume as seen in vitamin B_{12} deficiency and raised erythrocyte sedimentation rate in myopathies.
- Serum electrolytes and glucose: hypokalaemia can cause weakness, and disorders of calcium can lead to muscle spasms and tetany.
- Liver function tests: chronic alcohol excess and malnutrition.
- Thyroid function tests: hypothyroidism can present with weakness.

- Serum creatinine kinase: muscle damage and disease result in a raised serum creatinine kinase.

Urinalysis

Glycosuria is often seen in polyneuropathies and diabetes which can present with muscle weakness. A raised level of Bence-Jones protein is suggestive of myeloma which can present acutely with cord compression secondary to a fracture.

X-rays

The use of X-rays will largely be determined by the history and examination. In the case of trauma to the spine or limbs with secondary nerve involvement and subsequent weakness, X-rays are often valuable at identifying injury.

Computerised tomography

Computed tomography (CT) scanning allows greater assessment, particularly of the bony structure of the spine and the intracranial space. It is often enhanced by the use of intravenous contrast. It is useful for detecting intracranial haemorrhage following trauma or as a cause of stroke and for identifying space-occupying lesions such as tumours or abscesses. It is also useful in the assessment of acute spinal injuries with damage to the spinal cord.

Magnetic resonance imaging

Magnetic resonance imaging (MRI) has proven very useful in the assessment of intracranial lesions and muscle pathology. It has advantages over CT in the ability to differentiate white matter from grey matter in the brain, the ability to image spinal nerve roots and the absence of harmful radiation. Intramuscular lesions such as tumours and abscesses are also well seen on MRI.

Electromyography and nerve conduction studies

These are the investigations of choice for peripheral nerve lesions. Conduction of a signal can be tested either through a muscle (electromyography, useful in assessing myopathic conditions) or along a nerve, as in the case of carpal or cubital tunnel syndrome.

Biopsy

When a tissue diagnosis is required, a biopsy can be taken from the area thought to be the cause of the muscle weakness. In the case of intracranial pathology, a brain biopsy can be taken. This is common practice for the diagnosis of suspected tumours where CT guidance is often used. It can also be taken from the brain to diagnose inflammatory or degenerative brain disease such as the new variant Creutzfeldt–Jakob disease. When a peripheral polyneuropathy is suspected, a nerve biopsy can help in diagnosis. In these cases, a biopsy can be taken from the sural nerve of the leg. For cases of myopathies, a muscle biopsy can be taken from the skeletal muscle in the arm or the leg.

Summary

Muscle wasting and weakness is a common sign in musculoskeletal medicine. The causes are numerous but are often differentiated by a thorough history and examination. In the case of trauma, the underlying cause is often relatively obvious. However, in the rarer polyneuropathies, the cause is often hard to find, and special investigations are required. Muscle weakness and wasting should not be ignored, as it often represents serious underlying pathologies, some of which, such as malnutrition or chronic alcohol excess, are imminently treatable.

PAINFUL JOINTS

Pain, and the perception of pain, is a complex interplay of physiological and psychosocial signals. It is a common presentation and a common finding in both the history and the examination of a patient. When taking a history, it is very important to gather as much information about the pain as possible. This should include the following:

- site;
- radiation;
- intensity;
- duration;

- onset;
- character (for example sharp or dull);
- associated features (for example nausea or vomiting);
- exacerbating factors and
- relieving factors.

Often, the cause of the pain can be identified through a thorough history and examination. Investigations should serve to prove or refute the differential diagnosis made on the basis of the history and examination.

Causes of a single painful joint
Trauma
Septic arthritis
Local malignant deposits
Osteoarthritis
Crystal arthropathies

Causes of multiple painful joints
Rheumatoid arthritis
Reactive arthritis
Seronegative arthritis
Postviral arthritis
Osteoarthritis

Generalised musculoskeletal pain
Pain affecting multiple joints is known as polyarthritis and is often a manifestation of a systemic, inflammatory arthritis. Inflammatory arthropathies are characterised by synovial inflammation.

Rheumatoid arthritis
- Chronic systemic symmetrical polyarthritis of unknown cause, characterised by inflammatory synovitis affecting mainly peripheral joints, as seen in the hands in Figure 6.5.
- More common in women than men with a slight familial tendency.

- Presentation is variable but often with swollen, painful small joints of the hands and feet, often worse in the morning. This progresses to affect large joints.
- There is often progressive deformity of affected joints due to the destructive synovial inflammation.
- Can also present with extra-articular manifestations such as pericarditis, lung fibrosis, anaemia and weight loss.

Reactive arthritis
- Acute, asymmetrical, lower limb arthritis usually occurring within a couple of weeks of an infection elsewhere.
- Occurs following an episode of gastrointestinal infection or a sexually transmitted disease.
- Often associated with uveitis (inflammation affecting the eye) or urethritis (inflammation affecting the urethra).
- If occurring together, uveitis, urethritis and arthritis are referred to as Reiter's disease.

Seronegative arthritis
- Group of disorders affecting the spine and other joints that tend to occur in families.
- Similar in presentation and histology as rheumatoid arthritis but lacking in the presence of the rheumatoid factor.
- Ankylosing spondylitis affects young adults and presents with sacroiliitis and low-back pain in the late teenage/early 20s, long before the onset of the typical curvature of the upper spine.
- It occurs in both men and women, though men present with severer symptoms.
- It can affect the eyes and the joints of the ribs, causing anterior chest pain.
- Peripheral, mostly large joints can be affected.
- Psoriatic arthritis is a type of arthritis affecting people who have psoriasis or those who have a family history of psoriasis.
- The skin manifestation may be mild, while the joint effects can be severely disabling.

Pain affecting a single joint

Trauma
Injuries to joints are usually in the form of a fracture that extends into the joint. Joints can also fill with blood, producing a haemarthrosis. Relatively inconsequential trauma may produce a haemarthrosis in those with a bleeding tendency such as haemophilia or those on warfarin. Joints with intra-articular ligaments such as the knee or the shoulder can be subject to ligamentous injuries.

Septic arthritis
This is an orthopaedic emergency. The sensitivity of the articular cartilage means that pus in the joint must be removed as soon as possible to prevent irreversible damage to the joint. Infection of a joint usually results from the spread of infection from elsewhere via the bloodstream (haematogenous). In children, because of the rich blood supply to the growing ends of bones, infective organisms can form a region of osteomyelitis which can spread via the joint capsule to infect the joint. Septic arthritis is often suggested by the history, but the examination reveals the diagnosis. The joint is hot, red and swollen, and the patient resists any movement of the joint.

Local malignant deposits
Tumours of the bone can be defined as primary (arising from the bone) or secondary (due to metastatic spread from a tumour elsewhere) and benign or malignant. Features from the history will often lead to the diagnosis. Patients with malignant tumours of the bone often complain of pain at or near a joint, particularly at night. Systemic features of weight loss, loss of appetite and general malaise also suggest the diagnosis. Tumours with a tendency to metastasise to the bone are the following:

Breast,
Bronchopulmonary,
Kidney,
Thyroid and
Prostate.

Osteoarthritis

Osteoarthritis is the most common disease affecting joints, with 65,000 hip replacements undertaken in the United Kingdom last year (National Joint Registry UK 2008). It can be primary, where no cause is identifiable, or secondary, when it develops to any other condition affecting joints. It is more common in women than men and most commonly occurs after the age of 50.

It is often diagnosed by the history alone. Pain is present, often at night, and is exacerbated by movement and activity. There is often swelling of the joint, and the range of movement is reduced because of not only pain but also the changes in the joint itself.

Any joint can be affected, but the commonly affected joints are the distal interphalangeal joints of the hands and feet, the hips (Figure 6.6), the knees and the spine.

Osteoarthritis is characterised by destruction of the normally smooth articular cartilage with subsequent narrowing of the joint space. As the cartilage is destroyed, the bone begins to articulate on another bone, causing pain. The other bone responds by developing accessory lesions to compensate for the abnormal load (osteophytes) and becomes hardened (subchondral sclerosis). All these features are identifiable on the X-ray, which remains the investigation of choice.

Crystal arthropathy

Broadly speaking, this can be divided into gout or pseudogout. Gout is characterised by the development of sodium monourate crystals within a joint because of hyperuricaemia. Gout is more common in obesity, high-protein diets, high alcohol consumption and diabetes. Crystal deposition can be precipitated by trauma, surgery, infection, starvation and renal failure. Pseudogout is caused by the deposition of calcium pyrophosphate crystals in cartilage, producing chondrocalcinosis.

Both gout and pseudogout present in a similar way with a sudden onset of pain, swelling and redness, commonly affecting the first metatarsophalangeal joint of the foot or another joint. Pseudogout tends to affect the knee or wrist joints. It can often be confused with cellulitis or septic arthritis because of the redness and swelling. In chronic states, gout can cause the development of gouty tophi, which are hardened areas of crystal deposits in the ear lobe, Achilles tendon and digits.

Specific joints

Pain in the hip
- Osteoarthritis.
- Traumas, for example fractured neck of the femur and common injury affecting elderly patients following a fall.
- Inflammatory arthritis, for example rheumatoid arthritis and ankylosing spondylitis.
- Transient synovitis: can occur following a viral infection, especially in children, but must be differentiated from septic arthritis.
- Trochanteric bursitis: inflammation of the trochanteric bursa that lies between the greater trochanter and the muscles of the outside of the hip.
- Avascular necrosis: can be due to a number of causes including steroids and excess alcohol consumption and in divers or deep-sea workers.
- Referred pain: pain in the hip can be referred from pathology affecting the spine. Alternatively, pathology affecting the knee may cause proximal hip pain.

Pain in the knee
- Osteoarthritis.
- Bursitis: the knee is surrounded by 13 bursae, all of which can become inflamed, leading to pain around the knee.
- Meniscal trauma: the menisci are semicircular cartilages that deepen the knee joint and act to absorb shock in axial loading. They can be damaged by twisting injuries often during sports.
- Cruciate ligament injury: the anterior and posterior cruciate ligaments are crossed ligaments in the knee that prevent forwards and backwards displacement of the femur on the tibia. They can be damaged in sports injuries, causing pain and instability.
- Ruptured popliteal or Baker's cyst: cystic swelling at the back of the knee which, if it ruptures, causes severe pain in the knee

and calf. It must be differentiated from a deep-vein thrombosis or arterial disease.
- Referred pain: pathology in the hip can present with pain in the knee. Examination of the knee must include a full examination of the hip.

Pain in the shoulder
- Osteoarthritis.
- Trauma: fractures of the proximal humerus are a common injury, particularly in the elderly, following a fall. Clavicle fractures are common in the younger age group, following a fall onto the outside of the shoulder. Anterior dislocation of the shoulder is a common injury, particularly during sports.
- Impingement syndrome/subacromial impingement: erosion of the rotator cuff tendons, particularly the supraspinatus tendon, due to an overhanging acromium; presents with pain in the shoulder, particularly with movements away from the body.
- Torn rotator cuff: can be acute, following trauma, or secondary to chronic erosion, particularly in the elderly and those with rheumatoid arthritis. Pain and loss of function in testing the rotator cuff reveal the diagnosis.
- Adhesive capsulitis: inflammation of the shoulder joint capsule causes pain and a reduced range of movement. It can occur following trauma or surgery and is more common in diabetes.

Pain in the back and neck
- Trauma: vertebral body fractures associated with osteoporosis are very common in elderly women. High-speed injuries can cause injuries to the spine with associated neurological impairment.
- Disc prolapse: acute protrusion of an intervertebral disc, causing pressure on the adjacent nerves or the spinal cord. It is characterised by pain and neurological impairment of the affected nerve root.
- Infection: haematogenous spread of infection can lead to abscess formation within the spine.

- Tumour: because of blood supply to the spine, it is a common site for metastatic deposits, particularly from prostatic carcinoma. Primary bone or haemopoietic tumours can present with pain in the back (e.g. multiple myeloma)
- Spinal stenosis: osteoarthritis of the facet joints of the spine and osteophyte formation can lead to narrowing of the spinal canal and nerve root entrapment.
- Ankylosing spondylitis.

History and clinical examination

Often, the cause of the pain can be identified through a thorough history and examination. Investigations should serve to prove or refute the differential diagnosis made on the basis of the history and examination.

When taking a history, it is very important to gather as much information about the pain as possible. This should include the following:

- site;
- radiation;
- intensity;
- duration;
- onset;
- character (for example sharp or dull);
- associated features (for example nausea or vomiting);
- exacerbating factors;
- relieving factors and
- whether the patient has had it before.

Specific investigations

Blood tests
- Full blood cell count: anaemia of chronic disease (normochromic, normocytic) is often seen in chronic rheumatological conditions. A raised white blood cell count is seen in septic arthritis. Thrombocytopaenia (low platelet count) is often seen in chronic inflammatory conditions.
- Inflammatory markers: erythrocyte sedimentation rate and C-reactive proteins are raised in inflammation and infection.

- Autoimmune profile: markers of immune mediators, directed against the body; can be elevated in rheumatoid arthritis, systemic lupus erythematosus, Sjorgen's syndrome and other autoimmune arthropathies.
- Bone profile: markers of calcium storage and homeostasis (for example alkaline phosphatase, serum calcium, parathyroid hormone).
- Protein electrophoresis: looks for proliferation of specific immunoglobulins elevated in myeloma.
- Serum urate: can be elevated in cases of gout.

Imaging studies
- Plain X-ray: first-line imaging study in cases of trauma and diagnostic investigation for osteoarthritis.
- MRI: useful for looking at the bone and soft tissue; first-line imaging technique for assessing the spine and for musculoskeletal tumours.
- Ultrasound: non-invasive imaging technique using high-frequency sound waves; useful for assessing soft tissues including tendons and muscles and for measuring the flow of blood.
- Bone scintigraphy: utilises the uptake of a radioactive dye by the bone; uptake is increased in areas of high bone activity such as an infection, an inflammation or a tumour.

Joint aspiration
Joints contain synovial fluid secreted by the lining membrane of the joint that acts as a lubricant for the joint. Fluid can accumulate in the joint, which can usually be aspirated with a needle and syringe with the patient awake. The fluid may be of the following:

- Blood: in cases of trauma, particularly in patients in hypocoagulable states (for example on warfarin).
- Serous fluid: in exacerbations of osteoarthritis, the joint can become filled by inflammatory fluid. This must be differentiated from infectious fluid.
- Pus: in cases of septic arthritis, the joint can quickly fill with pus, causing intense pain, swelling and warmth at the joint.

The fluid aspirated from the joint can be grown to reveal the causative organism.
- Crystals: in cases of crystal arthropathy, the joint can become distended with inflammatory fluid rich in crystals (either urate or pyrophosphate). The diagnosis is made by studying these crystals' reaction to light under a microscope.

DEFORMITY

The term 'deformity' can be defined as a distorted shape or form; it derives from the Latin word *deformitas* meaning mis-shapen.

Musculoskeletal problems often culminate in the development of a deformity, commonly at a joint. Non-traumatic causes of deformity are often insidious in onset with a progressive change in the appearance or the alignment of a limb or part of a limb. Because of the precise biomechanical nature of the limbs, deformity is seldom the presenting complaint and is often either the cause or the effect of pain. Deformity, like muscle wasting, is a sign of an underlying condition and is often multifactorial.

Causes

As with many signs in medicine, the causes of deformity are broadly divided into congenital and acquired.

Congenital causes of deformity

The limb buds of the developing embryo appear at 4 weeks, gestation. The developing limb bud has all the constituents of the developed limb, including the muscle, nerve, bone, skin and blood vessels. The bones themselves develop from cartilage with segmentation to form the joints. Bones of the limbs develop by ossification of the primitive cartilage from primary ossification centres at the centre of long bones. Secondary ossification centres develop at the end of limb bones towards the end of gestation and in early infant life. It is therefore possible to age a child by the appearance of the secondary ossification centres.

Abnormal limb development

Abnormalities of limb development, resulting in deformity, can be classified into seven groups (Swanson 1976):

- failure of formation, for example Fibular deficiency;
- failure of separation, for example radio-ulnar synostosis;
- duplication, for example polydactyly (multiple digits);
- overgrowth, for example macrodactyly (large digits);
- undergrowth, for example hypoplastic digits;
- congenital constriction band syndrome, for example amniotic bands;
- generalised skeletal abnormalities, for example achondroplasia.

Along with these conditions, there are the disorders associated with the confined space in which the foetus develops. These disorders are predominantly self-correcting but alarming for parents at the time of birth. Developmental dysplasia of the hip may be associated with the constriction of the foetus *in utero*. This, of course, is seldom self-correcting and can require complex corrective surgery, depending on the severity of the dysplasia.

Trauma to the developing skeleton

Paediatric trauma represents an entity distinct from adult trauma. While many of the injuries are similar, the methods of treatment are often poles apart. Because of the development of the skeleton, paediatric injuries heal far more quickly in children than in adults. Children are able to tolerate degrees of deformity far greater than in adults, as the developing skeleton will grow out the deformity over time. The developing skeleton is also prone to injuries that do not occur in adults because of the presence of secondary growth centres and the physes.

Injuries to the physis were classified by Salter & Harris in 1963 (Figure 6.7).

Type I and II injuries require little intervention, unless severe angulation occurs, and rarely result in growth deformity. Types III, IV and V are less common but require surgical intervention

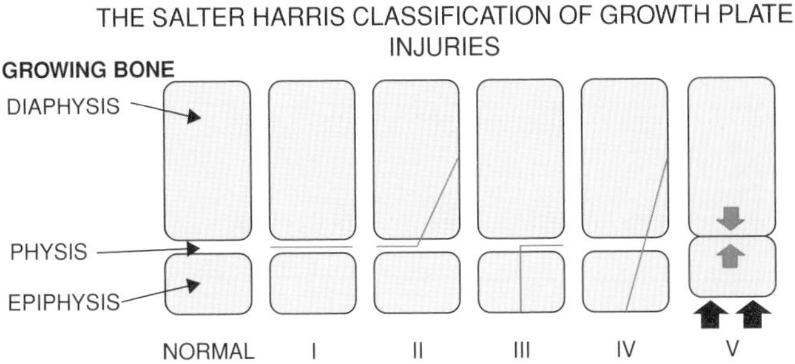

THE SALTER HARRIS CLASSIFICATION OF GROWTH PLATE INJURIES

GROWING BONE

DIAPHYSIS

PHYSIS

EPIPHYSIS

NORMAL   I   II   III   IV   V

Figure 6.7   Salter–Harris classification.

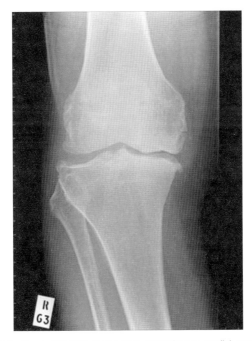

Figure 6.8   Varus deformity of the knee secondary to medial compartment osteoarthritis.

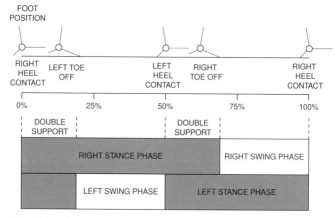

Figure 6.9   The normal gait cycle.

to restore the articular surface. Because the injury crosses the physis, there is a higher incidence of growth disturbance.

Acquired causes of deformity

- Trauma: deformity that is obvious and is associated with injury. Injuries to joints require anatomical reduction of the joint surface to prevent long-term deformity and progressive joint degeneration.
- Infection: chronic osteomyelitis can result in progressive destruction of bone and secondary deformity.
- Neoplasm: bone and soft tissue tumours can rapidly destroy the bone, leading to deformity. Soft tissue tumours (benign or malignant) often present with a lump that can be painless.
- Degenerative joint disease: can be localised to a single joint (for example osteoarthritis) or multiple joints (for example rheumatoid arthritis). Inflammatory arthropathies often have characteristic deformities such as those seen in the hands of patients with rheumatoid arthritis. In osteoarthritis of the knee, deformity is obvious because of either the varus or valgus angulation caused by the medial or lateral joint space destruction (Figure 6.8). Deformity of the first metatarsophalangeal joint is a common presentation in orthopaedic surgery.

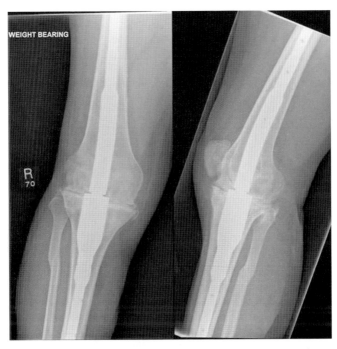

WEIGHT BEARING

R
70

Figure 6.10 Radiograph of the knee, showing arthrodesis in this case by an intramedullary nail. This knee had previously had a knee replacement, which had become infected.

This is caused by the valgus deformity of the great toe, causing the characteristic bunion.

- Deformity secondary to amputation: it is sometimes necessary to remove part or all of a limb. Currently in the United Kingdom, the most common indication for amputation of the leg is peripheral vascular disease. The indications for amputation are broadly divided into those where the affected limb is dead (for example because of a lack of blood supply secondary to chronic disease or trauma) or dangerous (for example because of severe soft tissue infections, such as necrotising fasciitis, or where removal of the limb is required to treat a tumour) or where the limb or part of the limb has become

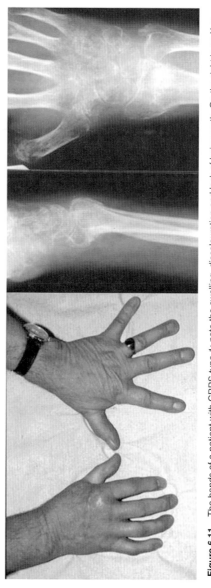

Figure 6.11 The hands of a patient with CRPS type 1; note the swelling, discolouration and lack of hair growth. On the right is an X-ray of a patient with CRPS type 1 affecting the hand; the woolly appearance of the bone is due to a relative osteopaenia.

a nuisance and limits the quality of life (for example removal of a digit in severe cases of Dupuytren's disease, chronic pain secondary to severe trauma or failed limb reconstruction in severe lower limb trauma).

History and clinical examination

As with all aspects of musculoskeletal disease, the cause is often revealed through a thorough history and examination. Specific questions from the history relating to deformity include the following:

- Time of onset: acute or chronic.
- Mechanism of deformity: is it related to a specific event or injury?
- Has the deformity been present since birth?
- Is the deformity progressive? Has it become worse?
- Associated symptoms: pain or loss of function.
- Adaptation and aids: many deformities can be compensated for with the use of walking aids, braces and shoe raises and inserts.
- Family history: does anyone else in the family have the deformity?
- Co-morbidities: other conditions resulting in deformity, for example diabetes and neurological conditions.

The clinical examination will be focused on the system highlighted from the history but, as with all medical examinations, should include a full general physical examination.

- Examine the affected area and the joints above and below.
- Clearly describe the nature of the deformity in terms of its site, severity and the plane in which it exists (valgus or varus, apex anterior or apex posterior, hyperextension or hyperflexion, rotational).
- Assess if the deformity can be passively corrected. Many deformities of the knee can be corrected because of laxity of ligamentous structures.
- Examine both active (what the patient can do themselves) and passive movements (what you can do with the patient relaxed).

- Examine the patient walking for lower limb deformities.
- Full neurological examination of both central and peripheral nerves.
- General examination for systemic diseases manifesting with deformity.

Specific investigations

The cause of the deformity is often apparent from the findings of the history and examination. If special investigations are required, these should be focused to the suspicions raised by the above-mentioned findings.

- Simple investigations
  - (1) Blood tests: these should be directed towards identifying a systemic cause of a progressive deformity, for example diabetes.
  - (2) Plain radiography: anteroposterior and lateral radiographs of the deformity the joints above and below. It is vital that radiographs are obtained in two plains, as some deformities are only visible in one plain and can therefore easily be missed.
- Special investigations
  - (1) CT and MRI: these may be required for two reasons – firstly, to image the central nervous system to identify a neurological cause of the deformity and, secondly, to image the deformity itself. This is often necessary for preoperative planning before corrective surgery.
  - (2) Nerve conduction studies: to identify a peripheral nervous system cause of the deformity.
  - (3) Specific blood tests: looking for specific markers of disease, for example the rheumatoid factor.

LOSS OF FUNCTION

Introduction

Loss of function is defined as a reduction in the complete actions or movements of the body or part of the body that were previously possible. As suggested, it is a temporal characteristic and as such can be acute or chronic and permanent or reversible. Causes of loss of function are seldom singular and are often the result of a complex interplay of not just anatomical but also psychological pathology. This is an aspect that must never be underestimated, as, all too often, it is easy to attribute a patient's symptoms and signs, or lack thereof, to a psychological cause. This is often as real as any anatomical deformity leading to a loss of function.

Causes of a loss of function

Gait abnormalities
Gait is the characteristic pattern by which the patients propel themselves, and its analysis is a vital part of the examination. It must always be assessed unaided, as subtle changes in gait can be masked by the use of a walking aid or articles on which the patient may lean. The normal gait is complex and relies on the interplay between the central nervous system and multiple joints including the spine, hips, knees and feet. The ability to walk relies not least on the perception of the world around us, and therefore, blindness may affect the way a person reacts to their surrounding environment. The body's ability to know where its limbs are is no accident; indeed large parts of the brain are involved solely in the perception of body position and the fine-tuning of signals from the brain required in moving the body. Abnormalities in any of these connections or motor centres will affect the way the body moves, causing characteristic movements.

The normal gait is a double pendulum, whereby the lead leg swings forward, articulating at the hip as the first pendulum. This strikes the ground at the heel of the foot. The foot then rolls to allow the body to swing over the foot as an inverted pendulum. Body weight is then transferred to the contralateral leg to allow the process to be repeated (Figure 6.9).

- Antalgic gait: commonly seen in pathology of the hip such as osteoarthritis; the patient leans towards the painful hip when bearing weight so as to reduce the weight put through the affected side. The stride length is also reduced.
- Trendelenburg gait: during the stance phase of the gait cycle, the pelvis is stabilised by the abductor muscles of the hip.

Pathology at the hip or weakness of these muscles will cause the pelvis to fall to the unaffected side. The result is that the body lurches towards the side of the pathology. Causes include osteoarthritis of the hip, superior gluteal nerve injury, L5 radiculopathy and polio.

- Scissor gait: this is most commonly seen in spastic cerebral palsy and is characterised by hypertonia of the legs, hips and pelvis, leading to a crouched stance, while excess adduction at the knees leads to crossing over of the legs during walking.
- Cerebellar ataxia: the cerebellum is an area of the brain involved in the integration of sensory perception, coordination and motor control. The gait of cerebellar ataxia is grossly uncoordinated and is due to damage to the cerebellum or its connections. It is demonstrated by Romberg's sign.
- Festinating gait: the patient moves with short, shuffling steps and finds difficulty in starting and stopping. It is characteristic of Parkinson's disease.
- Pigeon gait: in-toed gait often seen in children. It can be caused by rotational deformity of the hind foot, tibia or femur. The majority of cases resolve as the child grows.
- Steppage or high-stepping gait: this is caused by a loss of ankle dorsiflexion that requires the patient to bend the knee to allow the foot to be raised. Its causes include common peroneal nerve injury, Guillain–Barre syndrome, multiple sclerosis, nerve root lesions, peroneal muscle atrophy and polio.
- Myopathic gait: this is characterised by a waddling gait due to weakness of proximal muscles of the pelvic girdle. The patient uses circumduction of the hip to overcome the weakness of hip abduction. It is seen in pregnancy, hip dysplasia, spinal muscular atrophy and muscular dystrophy.
- Stomping or sensory ataxic gait: lack of proprioception causes the patient to walk with a high, stomping gait. It is seen in Freidrich's ataxia, tabes dorsalis, spinal cord disease, multiple sclerosis and peripheral neuropathy.

Pain

As previously described, pain at or about a joint will reduce the patient's desire to move the affected limb. Pain can be caused by a number of pathologies, but osteoarthritis is a common painful orthopaedic condition leading to loss of function. The loss of function seen in osteoarthritis is essentially a protective mechanism, whereby the stiffness of a joint prevents movement, the action which precipitates pain (Figure 6.10). The end stage of osteoarthritis is ankylosis, whereby the joint essentially fuses itself. This prevents movement of the joint and therefore, while significantly disabling, is often painless.

Trauma
There is often a loss of function following trauma, either due to the injury or secondary to the treatment. Prolonged immobilisation in a cast results in ligamentous and capsular shortening and subsequent joint stiffness. Trauma to joints results in stiffness at the joint and subsequent loss of function. Amputation secondary to trauma will carry with it a significant loss of function due not only to the anatomical loss but also to the psychological impact it has on the individual.

Complex regional pain syndrome
Complex regional pain syndrome (CRPS) is a chronic, severely disabling condition of unknown aetiology and uncertain pathophysiology, characterised by severe pain, swelling and changes in the skin (6.11). It is divided into type 1 (reflex sympathetic dystrophy, Sudeck's atrophy), where no identifiable nerve lesion is seen, and type 2 (causalgia), where symptoms are secondary to a peripheral nerve lesion. CRPS usually occurs following an injury including surgery. Symptoms often spread from the site of the injury and can involve the whole limb. Symptoms include burning pain and swelling. Trophic changes affecting the skin and nails include abnormal sweating, dry skin, abnormal and brittle nail growth and changes in the pattern of hair growth. CRPS can also affect the underlying bones with severe cases, causing features similar to osteoporosis. The joints become stiff and tender, and movements can be extremely painful.

History and clinical examination
As with all aspects of musculoskeletal disease, the diagnosis is often made following a full history and clinical examination.

Often, the cause can be localised to a single joint or limb, but the loss of a function can be multifactorial. Therefore, following a system-specific history and examination, a full general enquiry should be performed. Specific questions relating to a loss of function include those on the following:

- timing of onset – acute or chronic;
- duration of symptoms;
- rapidity of decline in function;
- what the patient can and cannot do;
- associated symptoms, for example pain, stiffness and deformity;
- how the patient accommodates for the deformity;
- co-morbidities and
- general medical enquiry including family and social history.

Specific aspects of the examination relate to the function that has been lost. Assessment of the gait, in particular, can reveal all that is needed to make the diagnosis. As with all musculoskeletal examinations, a thorough assessment of the joints above and below is always required. The examiner must always assess the peripheral nervous system and the vascular supply of the affected area.

Specific investigations

Investigations into a loss of function will be directed by the history and examination and will be composed of those detailed earlier. Loss of function secondary to musculoskeletal pathology is often best assessed using plain radiography and MRI. Neurological conditions presenting to an orthopaedic surgeon tend to arise from spinal pathology and are best assessed using MRI and nerve conduction studies.

REFERENCES

National Joint Registry Centre, Hemel Hempstead. http://www.njrcentre.org.uk/njrcentre/Default.aspx.

Swanson, A.B. (1976) A classification for congenital limb malformations. *Journal of Hand Surgery* **1**, 8–22.

Salter, R.B. & Harris, W.R. (1963) Injuries involving the epiphyseal plate. *Journal of Bone and Joint Surgery* **45**, 587–622.

Clinical Diagnosis of Symptoms Associated with the Genitourinary System

7

Dev Mittapalli and Dev Mohan Gulur

LEARNING OUTCOMES

At the end of this chapter, the reader will be able to discuss the clinical diagnosis of the following symptoms associated with the genitourinary system:

❏ anuria and oliguria,
❏ polyuria,
❏ urethral discharge,
❏ dysuria,
❏ incontinence,
❏ scrotal swelling,
❏ urinary retention and
❏ gynaecomastia.

ANURIA AND OLIGURIA

Anuria and oliguria are symptoms of different stages of acute renal failure (recently termed as Acute Kidney Injury, AKI). The normal urine output in a healthy human is 0.5–1 mL/kg/h, which in a 70-kg man roughly is 1.5 L/day. Oliguria is defined as decreased urine production of less than 400 mL in 24 h, and anuria is defined as complete absence of urine production for at least 12 h (some text books describe anuria as urine production less than 100 ml per 24 hours). It is a sign and symptom

Clinical Diagnosis, 1st edition. Edited by Phil Jevon.
© 2011 Blackwell Publishing Ltd.

Table 7.1 Causes of renal failure.

Pre-renal	Renal	Post-renal
Hypovolaemia Haemorrhage Hypoxia Heart failure (cardiogenic shock) Sepsis Dehydration	Acute glomerulonephritis (streptococcal throat infection, systemic lupus erythematosus, rhabdomyolysis) Acute tubular necrosis (shock, antibiotics, chemotherapeutic drugs) Acute interstitial nephritis (NSAIDs, diuretics, antibiotics)	Calculus in the urinary tract Cancers of the urinary tract Prostate cancer (most common cause in men) Iatrogenic (accidental ligation) Retroperitoneal fibrosis

(Sources: Llewelyn *et al*. 2009 and Raftery *et al*. 2010.)

of renal failure, which is an end result of various insults (see Table 7.1) to the kidneys. Oliguria is the beginning of renal failure, and anuria represents established renal failure. It is important to rule out blocked catheter before diagnosing anuria in a catheterized patient.

Causes
The causes for renal failure can broadly be divided into three main categories: pre-renal (related to blood supply to the kidneys), renal (intrinsic damage to the kidneys) and post-renal (obstruction to the urinary tract; Table 7.1). Urine production depends upon renal perfusion. Hypoxia, along with hypovolaemia, impedes renal perfusion and precipitates the renal failure (Llewelyn *et al*. 2009 and Raftery *et al*. 2010)

History and clinical examination
A detailed history to elicit the cause of renal failure should be sought. A history of diabetes, hypertension, pre-existing renal disease and medications like diuretics, non-steroidal anti-inflammatory drugs (NSAIDs) and angiotensin-converting enzyme inhibitors should be obtained. Family history of renal stones or pre-existing renal calculus and hypercalcaemia indicate post-renal failure. General features like poor appetite,

weight loss and the presence of haematuria suggest malignant pathology.

Associated clinical features include the following:

- Fever: if present, suggests infective pathology or sepsis.
- Pain: especially loin to groin pain is seen in patients with ureteric/renal stones.
- Haematuria: may be due to infection, renal stones or malignancy; it should be thoroughly investigated.

Oliguria in trauma and post-operative patients, unless proven otherwise, is due to hypovolaemia, and fluid replacement is the mainstay of treatment. These patients respond well to a fluid challenge. However, care should be taken not to overload the patient, especially those elderly who have a cardiac history. In anuria, where renal failure is well established, fluid balance should be monitored meticulously, as these patients are generally overloaded. In post-renal failure, obstruction should be relieved urgently.

As with any examination, thorough physical examination is necessary in patients presenting with oliguria or anuria. General examination may reveal dehydration, despite fluid retention, and confusion secondary to uraemia. These patients are usually critically ill and need thorough examination of all the systems. Depending on the aetiology, the findings may vary from simple dehydration to severe shock.

Specific investigations

- Urea and electrolytes (U&Es): blood urea is raised; serum creatinine is also raised and is a better guide of renal function, as it is unaffected by upper gastrointestinal (Upper GI) bleed, dehydration or liver disease. Raised serum potassium is one of the important indicators for dialysis. Serum sodium is reduced.
- Full blood count: haemoglobin may be low because of haemorrhage or anaemia. Raised white blood cells indicate infection.
- Liver function tests: deranged in case of hepato-renal syndrome.
- Specific gravity of urine: raised in pre-renal oliguria, as urine is concentrated, whereas in renal oliguria it is stable at 1010.

- Osmolality: increased in pre-renal oliguria because of urinary concentration (twice that of the plasma), but in renal oliguria it is equal to plasma osmolality.
- Microscopy: cells and casts present in renal oliguria.
- Electrocardiogram: broad QRS complexes, tall peaked T waves, ST depression and flat P waves may indicate hyper-kalaemia.
- Kidney, ureter and bladder X-ray: a simple and easily accessible tool for evaluation of stones.
- Intravenous pyelogram/urogram: a simple and easy test to assess obstruction but cannot be done in the presence of deranged renal function.
- Ultrasound scan of the renal tract: a useful and non-invasive test, especially in assessing renal and post-renal oliguria.
- Computerised tomography (CT) urogram: more accurate in assessing the kidneys, ureters and bladder.
- Magentic resonance imaging (MRI) scan: usually used in staging of prostate cancer.
- Nuclear medicine: dynamic isotope renography using mercaptoacetylglycine (MAG) and static isotope renography using dimercaptosuccinic acid (DMSA) are very accurate in assessing upper urinary tract obstruction and renal function. Ethylenediaminetetraacetate clearance is the best way to measure glomerular filtration rate.

POLYURIA
Polyuria is defined as excessive production of urine in excess of 3 L/day (Reynard *et al.* 2006).

Causes
Causes of polyuria include the following (Llewelyn *et al.* 2009, Raftery *et al.* 2010):

- Uncontrolled or ill-controlled diabetes mellitus.
- Sudden relief of chronic urinary obstruction, that is, high-pressure chronic retention in elderly men and post-operative diuresis due to saline loading. The urine osmolality (solute load) is greater than 250 mOsm/kg.
- Polydipsia (increased thirst) or diabetes insipidus. Diabetes insipidus is a condition characterised by a lack of the

anti-diuretic hormone (ADH) secreted by the posterior pituitary gland. The ADH is responsible for concentrating urine so that excess fluid is not lost in the urine. Diabetes insipidus can be caused by posterior pituitary failure (central diabetes insipidus) or by drugs like lithium, which damage the ADH receptors in the kidney (nephrogenic diabetic insipidus). Psychogenic polydipsia is another condition where the patient has the habit of 'compulsive water drinking'.

- Physiological response in cold weather because the body does not lose water, which is compensated by the increased urination.
- Diuretics, for example furosemide and bendrofluazide, induce excessive fluid and salt loss. They are used in treating hypertension and congestive cardiac failure which is characterised by excessive fluid accumulation due to a failing heart.
- Diuretic beverages, for example tea and alcohol, can induce diuresis. Headache caused by a hangover after a drinking binge is due to dehydration the next morning.

History and clinical examination

A history of frequent visits to the toilet and passing light-coloured (dilute) urine, a history of diabetes mellitus and control with oral hypoglycaemics or insulin and psychiatric illness needing lithium medications and diuretics, are all important. Past medical history of problems like congestive cardiac failure should also be obtained. It is important to enquire about the patient's fluid intake, including alcohol and beverages like tea and coffee.

Infection in diabetes mellitus can cause poor control of blood sugar, leading to polyuria. Exposure to cold weather can increase urination. Increased dosage of diuretics in cardiac patients can precipitate diuresis.

Polyuria can limit the lifestyle and social functioning of the patient. Care should be taken in the management of these patients, and where dehydration is present, hospital admission and strict fluid balance are mandatory. Once dehydration is treated, further management should be tailored towards treating the cause.

Specific investigations
- Frequency volume chart (Bladder diary)
- Urine osmolality – to differentiate between solute and water dieresis
- Blood tests, for example blood glucose and U&Es
- Hormonal assays – to exclude pituitary tumour
- Radiological investigations – to exclude pituitary tumour

(Source: Raftery *et al*. 2010)

URETHRAL DISCHARGE

Urethral discharge is an abnormal secretion of a purulent/seropurulent (mixture of pus and blood) in the urethra. It may be painful or painless and may not be associated with urination.

Causes

Causes of urethral discharge include the following:

- Sexually transmitted diseases, for example gonorrhoea, chlamydial infection and syphilis, are a common cause of urethral discharge.
- Urethritis (inflammation of the urethra).
- Reiter's syndrome, which includes arthritis, conjunctivitis and urethritis and does not have an infective cause.
- Prostatitis can cause urethral discharge along with deep-seated pelvic pain. Men may also experience painful ejaculations with lack of orgasm.
- Urethral cancer can sometimes present as urethral discharge. The discharge generally tends to be bloody. The patient may also present with blood in his urine (haematuria). This is more common in smokers, exposure to industrial dyes and chemicals and chronic exposure to smoke. This will need further investigations with an urgent referral to the urology team for flexible cystoscopy, renal ultrasound and urine cytology.

History and clinical examination

A good history of the patient's sexual life is essential. The patient has to be reassured about the maintenance of confidentiality. The sexual history should include any recent change in sexual partners, multiple partners and recent un-protected intercourse. Sexual promiscuity is also an important factor.

Conditions like diabetes mellitus that depress the immune system, immunosuppressants like steroids and HIV can predispose patients to acquire infections more easily.

Clinical examination should include a general physical examination, abdominal examination, digital rectal examination and examination of the external genitalia including a scrotal examination in males and per vaginal examination in females (see Figure 7.1).

Specific investigations
- Swab of discharge: for microbiology, culture and senstivity.
- Midstream urine specimen: needs to be sent to the laboratory. The urine is cultured in the laboratory to check for the growth of micro-organisms.

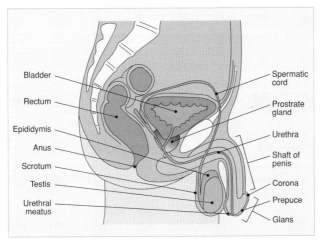

Figure 7.1 Male genitalia including scrotal contents. Reproduced from Adler M., *et al.* (2004) *ABC of Sexually Transmitted Infections*. 5th edn. Blackwell Publishing, Oxford; and adapted from the Sexually transmitted infections: history taking and examination CD published by the Wellcome Trust, 2003.

- Chlamydia polymerase chain reaction of the urine: performed to isolate chlamydiae.
- Flexible cystourethroscopy: an endoscopic examination of the urethra and the bladder. This is routinely performed under local anaesthesia. Biopsies can be taken if any suspicious areas are seen in the bladder or the urethra.
- Radiological investigations: may be needed in some cases.

DYSURIA

Dysuria can be defined as painful or difficult urination (derives from the Greek word *dus* meaning difficulty; Soanes & Stevenson 2006).

Causes

Dysuria is usually associated with a urinary tract infection (UTI). A UTI is defined as the presence of bacteria of more than 10^5 colony-forming units per millilitre of urine. UTI is usually caused by a bacterium, for example *Escherichia coli, Enterococcus, Klebsiella* or *Proteus*.

Precipitating factors

Women of reproductive age and children have a slightly increased risk of UTI. Elderly men with prostatic hypertrophy are predisposed to UTI because of residual urine in the bladder. These patients do not empty their bladder completely at the end of micturition. Patients with long-term catheters are also predisposed to have bacteria in the urine without causing inflammation of the urinary tract. Presence of stones in the kidney and bladder can increase the predisposition to UTI. Diabetes mellitus, steroids and immunosuppressants can decrease the immune status, increasing the risk of UTI.

History and clinical examination

The patient may experience the onset of painful or burning micturition, which may get progressively worse. A detailed history of the onset, duration and associated features is very important, as is a previous history of UTIs in case of recurrent UTIs.

Dysuria may be associated with fever, malaise, supra-pubic pain, frequency and small frequent voids. Bacterial colonisation of the bladder causes 'cystitis' and may cause ascending infection of the kidney, called 'pyelonephritis', which may make the patient systemically unwell, needing admission into the hospital for intravenous antibiotics and rehydration.

General physical and abdominal examination as with any other pathology should be undertaken. Scrotal and digital rectal examinations in men to estimate the size of the prostate and per vaginal examination in women are mandatory.

Specific investigations
- Midstream urine specimen: microscopy, culture and sensitivity.
- X-ray and ultrasound scan: if there is a suspicion of stones.
- Flow studies and post-micturition scans: in elderly men if there is a suspicion of prostatic obstruction.

INCONTINENCE
Incontinence is defined as the involuntary leakage of urine. It can be classified as follows:

- Stress incontinence: patients leak when the intra-abdominal pressure raises, for example on physical exertion or when they laugh, cough or giggle.
- Urge incontinence: patients have a sudden urge to pass urine. They end up leaking before they reach the toilet.
- Mixed incontinence: patients have a combination of stress and urge incontinence.

Causes
Stress incontinence is caused by a poor pelvic musculature, which can be due to a prolonged vaginal delivery with severe stretching of the muscles. It can also be secondary to pelvic trauma. Stress incontinence in men can be a complication of radical prostatectomy (open removal of the prostate for cancer).

Urge incontinence is usually due to an overactive bladder.

History and clinical examination
Patients are predominantly women. Patients with stress incontinence present with leakage of urine on suddenly standing up,

walking, laughing or coughing. They use a pad and find it very distressing. An obstetric history is very important to elicit details about previous childbirths. They generally have a history of prolonged vaginal delivery.

Patients with urge incontinence present with a history of rushing to the toilet but wetting themselves just before reaching the toilet.

Elderly men may present with bed-wetting and incontinence, which can be due to prostatic hypertrophy causing overflow incontinence. This is also called high-pressure chronic retention, and the treatment for this is either a long-term catheter or transurethral resection of the prostate (TURP).

Incontinence can be extremely embarrassing to the patient and severely affects the lifestyle. Patients need to carry pads all the time and change them regularly to get rid of the offensive odour. Young patients invariably have a low self-esteem because of the negative psychological impact.

A general physical examination and abdominal examinations are important. Per vaginal and speculum examination in women is essential to examine the urethra, assess the tone of perineal musculature and check for cystocele or rectocele. Patient can be asked to cough with the finger pressing the urethra onto the pubic bone to elicit a stress leakage.

Specific investigations
Urodynamics are the tests of choice. They may or may not involve injection of a dye into the bladder and X-rays (video urodynamics). These tests help to differentiate whether the incontinence is due to stress, urge or a combination of both.

SCROTAL SWELLING
Scrotal swelling is defined as abnormal enlargement of the scrotum.

Causes
Scrotal swelling can be caused by a local (testes and epididymis) pathology or as a part of generalised oedema. In some cases the aetiology is not clear (idiopathic scrotal oedema). A summary of causes is listed in Table 7.2.

Table 7.2 Causes of scrotal swelling.

Local pathology	As a part of generalised oedema	Miscellaneous
Hydrocele	Congestive cardiac failure	Idiopathic scrotal oedema
Inguino-scrotal hernia		
Epididymal cyst	Hypoalbuminaemia	Leukaemia
Epididymo-orchitis	Nephrotic syndrome	
Varicocele		
Spermatocele		
Testicular torsion		
Testicular tumours (seminoma, teratoma)		
Haematocele (trauma/surgery)		
Gumma of the testes		
Sebaceous cyst		
Carcinoma of the scrotal skin		

History and clinical examination

A detailed history and examination are crucial in evaluation of scrotal swelling. The following details should be obtained:

Age: primary hydrocele, epididymo-orchitis and malignancy of the testes are common in young adults, whereas secondary hydrocele occurs in the middle-aged.

Occupation: carcinoma of the scrotum is common in people working in the tar industry.

Swelling: check whether the swelling is unilateral or bilateral.

Exact site and size of swelling: this should be ascertained as it these will help in making diagnosis.

Mode of onset and duration: these provide an indication to the diagnosis. Sudden onset and short duration are seen in torsion and haematocele; long duration is seen in primary hydrocele and malignancy.

Progress of the swelling: slow in malignancy and a hydrocele and rapid in inflammatory conditions.

Any history of trauma: points towards the diagnosis of haematocele.

Other features like pain, fever and local skin changes as well as review of other systems are very important to make diagnosis. These are described next.

Associated signs and symptoms
- Pain: sudden-onset excruciating pain in a teenage/young adult patient might be due to testicular torsion, and immediate action should be taken. Pain is also common with epididymo-orchitis.
- Fever: usually indicates infective pathology but could be a reactive phenomenon in torsion or malignancy. Fever with night sweats is common in tuberculosis.
- Redness of scrotal skin: indicates inflammation.
- Weight loss, chest pain and dyspnoea: seen in advanced testicular cancer.

The key to scrotal swelling evaluation is to confirm if the swelling is purely scrotal by performing the 'getting above the swelling' test and then to establish the tissue of origin and the cause of the swelling. Testicular torsion is a urological emergency. Hence, any suspicion of testicular torsion warrants either emergency colour Doppler or scrotal exploration. Scrotal swelling associated with trauma also needs urgent action. Solid mass arising from the testes is most likely due to malignancy and needs urgent specialist referral. Epididymo-orchitis needs treatment with antibiotics for at least 2 weeks.

When undertaking a clinical examination of scrotum, it is important to

- ensure adequate light and exposure,
- examine the patient in a comfortable position and
- examine the opposite scrotum.

Clinical examination of the scrotum should include the following:

Inspection: check for the site, size, shape and number of swellings. Inspect for peristaltic movements and cough impulse, which is diagnostic of hernia. Check the skin over the scrotum and examine the penis.

Palpation: palpate the scrotum to confirm inspection findings as well as to determine the nature of the swelling. Check for temperature and tenderness, followed by the size, shape,

surface and consistency. Perform the following tests to define the nature of the swelling:

- Reducibility and cough impulse are signs of inguino-
  scrotal hernia.
- Getting above the swelling confirms that the swelling is
  scrotal.
- Indentation test – pitting oedema seen in cellulitis and
  nephrotic syndrome.
- Fluctuation is present in cystic swelling.
- Transillumination is positive in cystic swelling containing clear fluid (hydrocele, epididymal cyst). It is negative
  in swellings with thick fluid (pyocele, haematocele).
- Palpation of the testis, epididymis and spermatic cord:
  check whether the testis is palpable or not. If the testis is
  not palpable separate from the swelling, it is most likely
  hydrocele or pyocele or haematocele. If the testis is palpable, check whether the swelling is arising from the
  testis (testicular tumour) or the epididymis (epididymal
  cyst). Tenderness indicates infection, as does thickened
  epididymis.
- Examination of the opposite scrotum.
- Regional lymph nodes: the lymphatic drainage of the different parts of scrotum occurs separately to different regional lymph nodes. Check inguinal (scrotal skin), para-
  aortic (testes and epididymis) and left supra-clavicular
  (the testes indirectly drain here) lymph nodes.
- Rectal examination: in late-stage tuberculosis epididymi-
  tis, seminal vesicles may be involved (craggy, nodular
  seminal vesicles above the prostate).
- Other systems like the abdomen and the chest may reveal
  the focus of tuberculosis or metastatic deposits.

Key features of some of the important scrotal swellings are
described in Table 7.3.

Specific investigations

Blood tests: raised white blood cells in inflammatory lesions,
Venereal Disease Research Laboratory test in syphilis and
tumour markers for testicular tumours (alpha feto-protein,

Table 7.3 Causes of scrotal swelling together with associated clinical features.

Scrotal swelling	Important features
Hydrocele	Cystic swelling, can get above the swelling, transillumination positive, the testes not palpable
Haematocele	History of trauma, bruising, firm to hard, transillumination negative, may be tender
Pyocele	Cystic swelling, may be firm; signs of infection like erythema, tenderness present
Varicocele	Dilated, tortuous veins feel like 'bag of worms', non-tender, decompress on lying down
Inguino-scrotal hernia	Cough impulse positive, cannot get above the swelling, the testes palpable separate from swelling
Tumour	Hard, solid lesion, non-tender, the testes may be palpable separately
Torsion	Excruciating pain, sudden onset, exquisitely tender, the testes may lie horizontally, the epididymis usually not swollen
Epididymo-orchitis	Sever pain, both the testes and the epididymis swollen and tender, lifting the testes relieves pain
Epididymal cyst	Cystic swelling arising from the epididymis, brilliantly transilluminable, the testes can be felt separately
Sebaceous cyst	Fixed to the skin, smooth surface with punctum
Swelling secondary to generalised disease	Usually bilateral, pitting oedema, associated with oedema elsewhere, the testes and epididymis can be palpable separate from swelling

beta human chorionic gonadotropin, lactate dehydrogenase).

Urine: urinalysis and culture aid in the diagnosis of infective scrotal swellings.

Fluid analysis: aspirated fluid from cystic swellings helps in diagnosis. Clear water-like fluid – epididymal cyst. Straw-coloured fluid – hydrocele. Blood-stained fluid – haematocele. Purulent fluid– pyocele. Barley-water-like fluid – spermatocele.

Urethral smear: urethral discharge collected after prostatic massage may help in the diagnosis of gonorrhoea and chronic prostatitis.

Ultrasound scan: this is a non-invasive test and is the first radiological investigation for scrotal swellings. It differentiates solid lesions from cystic lesions.

Doppler ultrasound scan: it may be of value in testicular torsion to check for blood supply of the testis, but in doubtful cases the scrotum should be explored surgically.

Chest X-ray: usually to check metastatic disease and also any focus of infections like tuberculosis.

CT scan: used as a staging tool for malignant scrotal lesions.

RETENTION OF URINE

Retention of urine is defined as the inability to pass urine. It can be acute or chronic. Acute urinary retention occurs suddenly in a previously healthy urinary tract but can also occur as a part of acute-on-chronic retention. The retention can be due to either obstruction in bladder outflow or neurological disturbances. The bladder outflow obstruction can be due to various pathologies in the urinary tract from the urinary bladder to the external urethral meatus or external compression. An understanding of the urinary tract anatomy is important in retention of urine (Table 7.4).

Causes

Causes of retention of urine are listed in Table 7.4.

Table 7.4 Causes of urinary retention.

Urinary bladder	Urethra	External compression	Neurological
Calculus (stone) Tumour (benign or malignant)	Stricture Urethritis Calculus	Benign prostate hypertrophy or prostate cancer	Spinal injury Old age/senile atonic bladder
Blood clot (clot retention)	Phimosis Carcinoma	Faecal impaction Retroverted gravid uterus	Post-operative (especially after spinal anaesthesia)
		Rectocele and cystocele	Multiple sclerosis
			Drugs like anticholinergics

History and clinical examination

Urinary retention is one of the common cause for acute urological admissions. A detailed history is paramount in evaluation of urinary retention. Obtain the time of onset and the duration of symptoms as well as associated features. Acute urinary retention is usually sudden in onset; the patient is anxious with a full bladder and has spasmodic pain, but there are no obvious preceding symptoms. On the other hand, chronic urinary retention is painless; the patient is unaware of a distended bladder, and usually there will be a history of long-standing difficulties in voiding, especially in males.

Associated signs and symptoms include the following:

- Haematuria: the presence of frank haematuria points towards clot retention.
- Dysuria and frequency are due to UTI.
- Recurrent UTIs and poor stream indicate urethral stricture.
- Prostatism and lower urinary tract symptoms are usually due to benign prostatic hypertrophy.
- Weight loss and bone pains may be due to prostate cancer.

Urinary retention is more common in males and is usually due to prostate hypertrophy (either benign or malignant). These patients may have symptoms of poor stream, difficulty in voiding, sensation of incomplete voiding and urgency and frequency of micturition, including nocturia (need to wake up and pass urine at night usually more than once). All these features are generally described as 'prostatism' or 'LUTS' (lower urinary tract symptoms). Nocturia should not be confused with nocturnal enuresis where urine is passed unintentionally and is common in children but can occur in elderly patients having chronic retention with overflow. Chronic retention can be associated with chronic renal failure. These patients should be closely monitored following catheterisation for post-obstructive dieresis.

All the patients should undergo complete general physical examination including genital examination. Abdominal examination may reveal lower abdominal discomfort with suprapubic fullness and palpable bladder. Percussion is more sensitive in determining whether the urinary bladder is full or not.

However, it may be difficult to palpate the bladder in an obese patient; a bladder scan may be helpful. Common causes like constipation (faecal impaction) and enlarged prostate can be easily evaluated by per rectal examination and must be performed in all patients. Pelvic/per vaginal examination should also be performed, as external compression by pelvic pathology can cause retention.

Specific investigations
- Urinalysis: to screen for infection (leucocytes and nitrites) and haematuria.
- Urine culture: to confirm the infection.
- Urine cytology: may show malignant cells, warranting further investigations.
- Bladder scan: portable ultrasound to determine the volume of urine in the bladder. If post-voiding scan shows more than 100 mL, the patient is considered to be in retention. More accurate measure is if the residual volume is more than 40% of total volume i.e residual plus voided volume.
- Blood tests: may show raised inflammatory markers in infection. U&Es may be deranged, especially creatinine. Usually two thirds of renal function have to be damaged before the U&Es are deranged. Prostate-specific antigen should be done routinely especially in elderly patients.
- Cystoscopy: useful for both diagnostic and therapeutic purposes. It can diagnose urethral stricture or prostate hypertrophy. If there is bladder stone or blood clot, it can be extracted to relieve the obstruction.
- Urodynamics tests: these tests help to determine the functional (detrusor over/under activity) as well as obstructive causes of retention.
  (1) Urinary flow rate and peak flow are non-invasive and are easily done.
  (2) Bladder capacity and residual volume are important, as patients with chronic retention tend to have increased capacity as well as residual volume.
  (3) Other tests like bladder pressure measurement are invasive but can be useful in chronic retention.

- Radiological investigations
  (1) Retrograde cystogram/urethrogram helps in diagnosing urethral stricture as well as bladder pathologies like bladder stones and tumours.
  (2) Ultrasound scan is non-invasive and can identify bladder lesions.
  (3) CT and MRI scans are more sophisticated and are used as staging tools for urological cancers including prostate cancer.

GYNAECOMASTIA

Gynaecomastia, also known as gynaecomazia, is defined as 'hypertrophy of the male breast'.

Causes

Gynaecomastia is generally caused by either excessive oestrogens (female hormones) or suppression of androgens (male hormones). Some of the important causes are listed next.

- Congenital: neonatal gynaecomastia due to circulating maternal oestrogens and Kleine felter's syndrome.
- Iatrogenic: orchidectomy for prostate carcinoma, torsion testis or testicular tumours.
- Inflammatory: orchitis due to tuberculosis, syphilis, mumps and the like.
- Neoplastic: choriocarcinoma of the testes (excessive gonadotrophin production), ectopic hormone (oestrogen) production by bronchogenic carcinoma and adrenal and pituitary tumours.
- Drugs: for example digitalis, cimetidine, diuretics (spironolactone) and salbutamol.
- Hormonal therapy: oestrogens for prostate cancer.
- Cirrhosis of the liver.

History and clinical examination

A detailed history to elicit the cause of gynaecomastia is the key. Most often there is an aetiological factor, but in some cases like gynaecomastia in boys at puberty, the aetiology is unknown. Enquire about medication and a history of hormonal therapy.

Details of previous surgeries and infections like mumps and syphilis, which can affect the testes, are important. A history of liver disease is also important, as there is increased circulating oestrogen due to failure of its metabolism in the liver. These patients may have features of hepatic failure or portal hypertension like spider naevi and capute medusae.

The key in the management of gynaecomastia is to determine the cause, and most cases need avoiding/removing the aetiological agent, and reassurance is all that is needed. However, any suspicion of malignancy should warrant thorough investigation and specialist referral for further management, as breast cancer in males is quite aggressive.

Gynaecomastia should be assessed carefully by triple assessment if there is any suspicion of malignancy. This includes clinical examination, radiological investigation and histological diagnosis.

Specific investigations

- Blood tests: to check for infections. Also perform special tests for specific infections like mumps and tuberculosis. Liver function tests should be done to check for liver failure.
- Mammography or ultrasound scan: in case of malignancy.
- Excisional biopsy: for diagnostic and therapeutic purposes.
- Palpation and examination of the testes: to exclude malignancy as the cause.

REFERENCES
Dawson, C. & Whitfield, C. N. (2006) *ABC of Urology*, 2nd edn. BMJ Books, London.
Llewelyn, H., Ang, H., Lewis, K. *et al.* (2009) *Oxford Handbook of Clinical Diagnosis*, 2nd edn. Oxford University Press, Oxford.
Raftery, A., Lim, E. & Ostor, A. (2010) *Differential Diagnosis*, 3rd edn. Elsevier, London.
Reynard, J., Brewster, S., & Biers, S. (2006) *Oxford Handbook of Urology*, 1st edn. Oxford Unoversity Press, Oxford.
Soanes, C. & Stevenson, A. (eds) (2006) *Concise Oxford English Dictionary*, 11th edn. Oxford University Press, Oxford.

8 Clinical Diagnosis of Symptoms Associated with the Ears, Nose and Throat

Dev Mittapalli

The aim of this chapter is to understand the clinical diagnosis of symptoms associated with the Ear, Nose and Throat (Otorhinolaryngology) system.

LEARNING OUTCOMES

At the end of this chapter, the reader will be able to discuss the clinical diagnosis of the following symptoms associated with the ears, nose and throat:

- ❏ dysphagia,
- ❏ deafness,
- ❏ sore throat and
- ❏ mouth ulcers.

DYSPHAGIA

The term 'dysphagia' can be defined as difficulty or discomfort in swallowing; it derives from the Greek words *dus* meaning 'difficult' and *phagia* meaning 'eat' (Soanes & Stevenson 2006). Other words that are synonymously used are aglutition, aphagia or odynophagia, even though there is a slight literal difference among them. The first two mean complete inability to swallow, whereas the last means painful swallowing (*odyno* = pain, *phagia* = swallowing). The other words worth mentioning

Clinical Diagnosis, 1st edition. Edited by Phil Jevon.
© 2011 Blackwell Publishing Ltd.

here, even though not related, are aphasia and dysphasia, which mean difficulty or inability in speech.

Swallowing has four stages:

- oral preparatory,
- oral,
- pharyngeal and
- oesophageal.

Causes

The causes of dysphagia can be broadly divided into pre-oesophageal, which includes oral and pharyngeal, and oesophageal causes. The oesophageal lesions can be in the lumen, on the wall or outside the wall. The causes are outlined next (Llewelyn *et al.* 2009, Raftery *et al.* 2010).

Pre-oesophageal (oropharyngeal)

(1) Oral phase: these are secondary to disturbances in mastication (trismus, fractured mandible), lubrication (xerostomia, radiotherapy) or mobility of the tongue (paralysis or tumours of the tongue). They can also be due to anatomical defects like cleft palate or lesions of mucosal ulcers.
(2) Pharyngeal phase: these are usually either obstructive lesions of the pharynx (tumours of the tonsil or pharynx or hypertrophic tonsils) or inflammatory conditions like acute tonsillitis, epiglottitis and quinsy (peritonsillar abscess). Paralysis of the soft palate, stroke and bulbar palsy can also interfere with swallowing, causing dysphagia.

Oesophageal

(1) Lumen: foreign body, oesophageal atresia, stricture and tumours, especially malignancies.
(2) Wall: achalasia, scleroderma and diffuse oesophageal spasm.
(3) Outside the wall: enlarged thyroid or cervical lymph nodes and tumours of the mediastinum.

History and clinical examination

The clinical presentation of dysphagia mainly depends on the aetiology. A detailed history is very important. The onset and progress of the dysphagia, along with associated features like weight loss and reflux symptoms, are important in the clinical diagnosis.

Sudden-onset dysphagia is seen in foreign body or impaction of food on a pre-existing stricture or malignancy. Progressive dysphagia for solids with a sensation of food sticking is seen in carcinomas and strictures. Dysphagia for solids more than liquids is seen in pharyngeal pouch (pharyngo-oesophageal pouch), xerostomia, post-cricoid web and globus hystericus (globus pharyngeus). Pharyngeal pouch will also cause regurgitation of undigested food with cough at night, halitosis and sensation of lump in the neck as well as bulge in the neck. Globus pharyngeus is a sensation of lump in the throat and is commonly associated with anxiety. Post-cricoid web is associated with severe iron deficiency.

Dysphagia more to liquids than solids is seen in neurological disorders like myasthenia gravis, motor neuron disease, achalasia and bulbar and pseudo-bulbar palsies. It is also seen in diffuse oesophageal spasm. Intolerance to acidic food and fruit juices is seen in ulcerative lesions.

The clinical examination should include general examination to find out the peripheral sign like anaemia, clubbing, weight loss, muscle weakness or hemiparesis, all of which can be of value to differentiate between neurological and malignant causes. Examination of the oral cavity, oropharynx and larynx helps to rule out most of the pre-oesophageal causes. Examination of the neck might reveal an enlarged thyroid. Examination of the chest and nervous system, including cranial nerves, is also important in assisting clinical diagnosis.

Specific investigations

The investigations should be tailored according to the aetiology of the dysphagia. Some of the important investigations are as follows:

- Blood tests: full blood cell count may reveal anaemia (Plummer–Vinson syndrome) or raised white blood cell count (inflammatory or infectious conditions). Serum proteins and albumin will determine patient's nutritional status. Abnormal thyroid function tests may point towards thyroid as the cause of dysphagia.

- Imaging studies: (1) The chest X-ray may show cardio-pulmonary or mediastinal lesions. (2) The lateral neck view will show any soft tissue shadows in the retropharyngeal space. (3) Barium swallow is very useful in the diagnosis of achalasia, strictures, oesophageal spasm and malignancy. (4) Videofluoroscopic swallowing study is the combination of barium swallow and fluoroscopic control and is valuable in the diagnosis of motility disorders. (5) A computed tomography (CT) scan gives more detailed information of the head, neck and chest, especially the mediastinum.
- Endoscopy: (1) Oesophago-gastro-duodenoscopy allows direct visualisation and biopsy of oesophageal and gastric lesions. (2) Fibre-optic endoscopic examination of swallowing is used in assessing pharyngeal swallowing.
- Manometry and pH monitoring: These are of value in patients with achalasia and reflux disease.
- Other tests like brochoscopy and angiogram may be of help if bronchial carcinoma or vascular anomalies are suspected.

The management of dysphagia mainly depends on the aetiology and is beyond the scope of this book. However, any suspicion of malignancy warrants urgent specialist referral. Patients with dysphagia, where there is a risk of aspiration (stroke), should be assessed by a speech and language therapist (SALT) before the initiation of oral feeding.

DEAFNESS
Deafness is defined as difficulty in hearing. It can be either conductive or sensorineural.

Causes

Conductive deafness
The causes of conductive deafness could be congenital or acquired.

(1) Congenital causes
- atresia of the external auditory canal,
- ossicular anomalies and
- absent oval window.

(2) Acquired causes
- External ear conditions
  Foreign body, wax;
  External otitis;
  Tumours of the external auditory canal.
- Middle ear conditions
  Fluid in the middle ear, for example acute suppurative otitis media;
  Tympanic membrane perforation, either infective or traumatic;
  Tumours of the middle ear;
  Fixation of the ossicle, for example otosclerosis;
  Blocked Eustachian tube.

Conductive deafness is usually caused by either obstruction in the external ear or perforation of the tympanic membrane. Bilateral progressive sensorineural loss is usually from degenerative ageing changes in the cochlea (presbyacusis). Unilateral progressive sensorineural loss is most often due to either Meniere's disease (disease of unknown cause, affecting the membranous labyrinth of the ear and causing progressive deafness and attacks of tinnitus and vertigo; Soanes & Stevenson 2006) or acoustic neuroma. Sudden sensorineural deafness is usually secondary to trauma. However, unilateral sudden hearing loss might be a sign of acoustic neuroma.

(Sources: Llewelyn *et al*. 2009 and Raftery *et al*. 2010)

Sensorineural deafness
The causes of sensorineural deafness can be either congenital or acquired.

(1) Congenital causes
- genetic causes like Down's syndrome and Michel's aplasia (absent inner ear);
- non-genetic causes like ototoxic drugs (streptomycin), viral infections (rubella), birth trauma and anoxia.

(2) Acquired causes
- infections of the labyrinth – viral or bacterial;
- trauma to the labyrinth or eighth cranial nerve;
- ototoxic drugs like gentamycin, ampicillin, furosemide and ibuprofen;
- Meniere's disease;
- acoustic neuroma;
- familial progressive sensorineural hearing loss.

(Sources: Llewelyn *et al.* 2009 and Raftery *et al.* 2010)

History and clinical examination

The history is very important to know the aetiology of the deafness. Ascertain the age of onset, whether unilateral or bilateral, whether stationary or progressive, any association with other conditions and involvement of other family members. Obtain any history of trauma, surgery and medications.

Associated signs and symptoms include the following:

- Fever indicates inflammation and is seen in acute suppurative otitis media.
- Pain is usually a sign of infection.
- Vertigo and tinnitus are usually seen in Meniere's disease along with sensorineural disease.

Clinical examination should be carried out mainly to find out the cause and type of hearing loss. Examination of the ear may reveal wax or foreign body. Otoscopy may show perforation of the tympanic membrane. Complete physical examination should be performed, as deafness can be associated with various syndromes. The two important bedside tests to differentiate conductive and sensorineural deafness are the Weber and Rinne tests. These tests are described in the next section.

Specific investigations

- Blood tests: white blood cells (WBCs) raised in infections, blood sugar and Venereal Disease Research Laboratory test, among others.
- Ear swab: send a swab from the affected ear(s) for bacteriology and culture if discharge/pus is evident.

Table 8.1   Interpreting the Rinne and Weber tests.

Hearing	Rinne test	Weber test
Normal	AC > BC bilaterally	Midline
Conductive deafness	BC > AC affected hear AC > BC normal ear	Lateralised to affected ear
Sensorineural deafness	AC > BC both ears	Lateralised to normal ear

AC, air conduction; BC, bone conduction.

- Tuning fork tests
  (1) Rinne test: normally, air conduction is better than bone conduction. The Rinne test is based on this principle. The vibrating tuning fork is placed 1 inch away from the external ear (Table 8.1). When the patients stop hearing, the tuning fork is immediately placed on the mastoid process. If the patient can still hear the vibrations, the Rinne test is negative.
  (2) Weber test: this test is useful in unilateral deafness. It is based on the principle of comparing bone conduction of both ears simultaneously. The tuning fork is placed in the middle of the vertex. It is heard equally on both sides in a person with normal hearing.

The interpretation of these two tests is shown in Table 8.1.

- Audiometry: pure tone audiometry, speech audiometry, impedance measurement and evoked response audiometry are sensitive and reliable.
- CT and magnetic resonance imaging scans: may be needed to evaluate deafness, especially lesions like acoustic neuroma.

SORE THROAT
'Sore throat' is a general term used to describe pharyngitis. Pharyngitis is an inflammation of the pharynx, which represents a variety of conditions like tonsillitis, tonsillopharyngitis or

nasopharyngitis. Pharyngitis can occur at any age, but the peak incidence is in children aged 5–10 years.

Causes

Pharyngitis can be acute or chronic. Acute pharyngitis is caused by various aetiological factors like viral, bacterial and fungal infections, whereas chronic pharyngitis is caused by chronic irritation secondary to various conditions. Viral causes are more common, but streptococcal infection can be very serious, as it can cause rheumatic fever and post-streptococcal glomerulonephritis. The causes of pharyngitis are listed next.

Acute pharyngitis

- Viral: rhinovirus, influenza and parainfluenza, measles and chicken pox, herpes simplex, infectious mononucleosis, cytomegalo virus and coxsackie virus.
- Bacterial: group A beta haemolytic streptococcus, diphtheria and gonococcus.
- Fungal: *Candida albicans*.
- Others: *Toxoplasma* and *Chlamydia*.

Chronic pharyngitis

- Persistent post-nasal discharge: secondary to rhinitis and sinusitis.
- Chronic irritants: for example chewing of tobacco and excessive smoking.
- Environmental pollutants: for example industrial fumes.
- Mouth breathing: may lead to dry mucosa, making it susceptible to infections.
- Atrophic pharyngitis: seen in patients with atrophic rhinitis.

History and clinical examination

The history is important to help make a clinical diagnosis. The following are important to note:

- onset, duration and severity;
- associated features, for example pain, fever and generalised malaise;

- presence of lymphadenopathy, either cervical or generalised;
- swallowing and breathing problems;
- previous episodes, including response to any treatment.

Unilateral pain may suggest peritonsillar abscess (quinsy). Associated hoarseness of the voice, especially in the elderly, may represent malignancy. Pharyngitis not responding to treatment should raise the suspicion of peritonsillar or retropharyngeal abscess.

There are no clear differentiating clinical symptoms or signs to ascertain the aetiology of pharyngitis. Laboratory tests might be helpful but not quick enough to start the treatment. However, some features apart from sore throat and painful swallowing may help to make a provisional diagnosis and initiate treatment. Viral pharyngitis presents with fever and cervical lymphadenopathy and lymphocytosis but normal leucocytes. Acute follicular tonsillitis presents with enlarged tonsils with white patches, cervical lymphadenopathy and leucocytosis. Infectious mononucleosis presents with enlarged tonsils, malaise, generalised lymphadenopathy and splenomegaly. Atypical lymphocytes are seen in WBCs. Candidiasis (oral thrush) is commonly seen in diabetics and immunocompromised patients, as well as recent antibiotic use. Examination reveals white plaques on the oral mucosa. Meningococcal infections will have features of meningitis (photophobia, headache and neck stiffness).

Clinical examination may reveal adenoid facies (half-open mouth, sleepy look and pinched-out nose). Inspection of the mouth and throat needs good light, a widely opened mouth and a spatula to depress the tongue. Asking the patient to say ah might help in visualisation of the pharynx, especially the tonsils. The pharynx may show granulations, purulent discharge or swelling (retropharyngeal abscess). Bimanual palpation with gloved fingers is crucial. Gentle compression of the anterior pillar of the tonsil with a spatula may express the pus in septic tonsillitis. Examination of all the lymph nodes, especially cervical nodes, and palpation of the abdomen for splenomegaly are important. Laryngoscopy should be performed to visualise the laryngopharynx.

Specific investigations
More often than not the treatment is initiated on the basis of provisional diagnosis, and further investigations are conducted to confirm the diagnosis. Some of the useful tests are listed next.

- Laboratory:
  (1) blood – WBCs in inflammatory conditions, haemoglobin, blood sugar (diabetes) and Venereal Disease Research Laboratory test (syphylis);
  (2) Mantoux skin test (tuberculosis);
  (3) biopsy for histological diagnosis of ulcer or lymph node;
  (4) microbiology – pus or discharge culture and sensitivity.
- Radiological imaging: the X-ray of the neck, especially the lateral view, is useful in retropharyngeal abscess.
- Endoscopy: laryngoscopy, direct or indirect or fibre-optic, is useful in visualisation of the larynx and obtaining pus swab or biopsy.

MOUTH ULCERS
An ulcer can be defined as an open sore on an internal or external body surface, caused by a break in the skin or mucous membrane that does not heal (Soanes & Stevenson 2006).

Causes
The causes of mouth ulcers can be broadly divided into infectious, traumatic, immunological (immune disorders and immunodeficiency), allergic and neoplastic. There are also some other rare causes. The causes are listed in Table 8.2.

History and clinical examination
The history should always start with patient demographics, that is, name, age and sex, as they will narrow the differentials in making the clinical diagnosis. The following details should be obtained in the history:

- location, onset, duration and progress of the ulcer;
- associated features, for example swelling, pain, fever and redness of mucous membranes (described in detail later);

Table 8.2 Causes of mouth ulcers.

(1) Infections
  - viral – herpes simplex, glandular fever and hand–foot–mouth disease;
  - bacterial – tuberculosis, syphilis, diphtheria, and Vincent's angina;
  - fungal – candidiasis.
(2) Immune disorders
  - Behcet's disease;
  - aphthous ulcers;
  - pemphigus vulgaris and lichen planus.
(3) Immunodeficiency: agranulocytosis, leukaemia, pancytopenia, neutropenia, diabetes and uraemia.
(4) Trauma
  - physical – cheek bite or ill-fitting dentures;
  - chemical – aspirin burn or phenol;
  - thermal – hot food and drinks and reverse smoking.
(5) Neoplasms
(6) Allergy: toothpaste, mouthwash and certain drugs, e.g. penicillins and sulphonamides.
(7) Vitamin deficiencies
(8) Miscellaneous: radiation mucositis, chemotherapy, etc.

- past medical and surgical history – similar episodes in the past (tuberculosis, syphilis and diabetes) and any previous operations particularly for cancers;
- personal history – enquire about eating habits (spicy and hot food) and smoking;
- family history – important especially in case of infective ulcers like tuberculosis.

The important associated signs and symptoms include the following:

- Pain: usually present in traumatic, dyspeptic and inflammatory ulcers. Pain is absent in primary chancre (syphilis) and early cases of malignant ulcer or growth. Pain may be present in late or advanced cases of cancer. Occasionally, pain may be referred from other sites having same innervations.
- Fever: usually present in inflammatory or infective ulcers.
- Constitutional symptoms: for example poor appetite and weight loss should raise the suspicion of malignancy.

- Impaired functions: for example difficulty in chewing and swallowing is common, especially in painful ulcers. Occasionally, speech might be affected if the pain is severe.

Ulcers can be classified as follows:

- Aphthous ulcers: recurrent, multiple, small superficial ulcers. They commonly occur in females and are related to stress.
- Viral ulcers: most commonly due to herpes simplex. These start as small vesicles and eventually rupture, forming multiple yellow ulcers with bright red margins. Regional lymph nodes are markedly enlarged.
- Syphilitic ulcers: usually painless and commonly occur on the lips (primary chancre), oral cavity (mucous patch and snail track ulcers) and tongue. These patients will also have genital lesions. Hence, sexual history and genital examination are crucial in diagnosing these lesions.
- Angular stomatitis: usually involves angle of the mouth and is due to vitamin B deficiency.

Mouth ulcers, more often than not, are a presentation of other systemic disease. Hence, clinical examination of mouth ulcers should be done systematically, that is, general examination followed by local examination including regional lymph nodes, as well as relevant systemic examination.

Good light and adequate exposure of the oral cavity are vital. Inspect the lips, cheeks, gums and teeth, palate, tongue and floor of the mouth. Examination of the oral cavity may reveal single or multiple ulcers, which may be superficial or deep. Palpate the lesions with a gloved finger; it is important to perform bimanual examination of the mouth lesions where necessary. Examine the cervical lymph nodes. Enlarged lymph nodes suggest either an inflammatory (painful) or a malignant (painless) cause.

Specific investigations
- Laboratory
  - (1) full blood count in inflammatory conditions;
  - (2) urine and stool culture for infections;
  - (3) pus for culture and sensitivity;
  - (4) sputum – for acid-fast bacillus in tuberculosis;

(5) biopsy – of value when the diagnosis is uncertain or there is suspicion of malignancy;

(6) immunological tests – might be needed in autoimmune disorders causing mouth ulcers.

- Radiological examinations: may show infective changes or infiltration of bones by cancerous lesions.
- Endoscopy: direct and indirect laryngoscope helps to visualise and diagnose lesions of the posterior third of the tongue and larynx.

REFERENCES

Llewelyn, H., Ang, H., Lewis, K., *et al.* (2009) *Oxford Handbook of Clinical Diagnosis*, 2nd edn. Oxford University Press, Oxford.

Raftery, A., Lim, E. & Ostor, A. (2010) *Differential Diagnosis*, 3rd edn. Elsevier, London.

Soanes, C. & Stevenson, A. (2006) *Concise Oxford English Dictionary*, 11th edn. Oxford University Press, Oxford.

Index

Clinical Diagnosis, 1st edition. Edited by Phil Jevon.
© 2011 Blackwell Publishing Ltd.